A Psychological Perspective of Health Personnel in Times of Pandemic

Juan Moisés de la Serna

Translated by Lauren Izquierdo

Tektime Editorial

2020

A Psychological Perspective of the Health Personnel in
Times of Pandemic

Prologue

Afterward the successful reception of the book entitled "Psychological Aspects in Times of Pandemic" where a number of issues from the perspective of psychological science are addressed, related to the impact of the appearance of COVID-19 on the lives of citizens, and afore readers´ insistent request for a text focused on health personnel, from there came this book.

The purpose of this, it is to offer updated information on the psychological aspects of who have been described as the battlefront against the advance of COVID-19 from a perspective of scientific psychology, for which reference will be made to the latest publications in this regard.

A rigorous and up-to-date vision of the contributions of the science of psychology told in a way that is accessible to everyone, with the aim of helping to understand the emotional impact of this situation on health personnel, as well as the present and future consequences of the same.

A Psychological Perspective of the Health Personnel in Times of Pandemic

Homage

Although it may be obvious, to speak of the health personnel is to speak of those who are in charge of health, whether physical or mental, and depending on how the distinction between professions and specialties within the health field is established in each country.

Perhaps the most notable difference in a hospital may be between health personnel versus non-health personnel, in this first case being the doctors, nurses and assistants; while within the category of non-health, management and administration personnel would be included, as well as support personnel such as orderlies, guards and even cleaning personnel, all of them essential for a more or less large health center to function conveniently.

The previous distinction is not trivial but has been brought up, because although the text focuses on health personnel in times of pandemic, it should not be forgotten that they can carry out their work thanks to the entire human team that is supporting them and collaborating with them; sometimes being "invisible" for patients and relatives, but as indicated before, they are of essential importance (@UNICEF_CLM, 2020) (see Illustration 1).

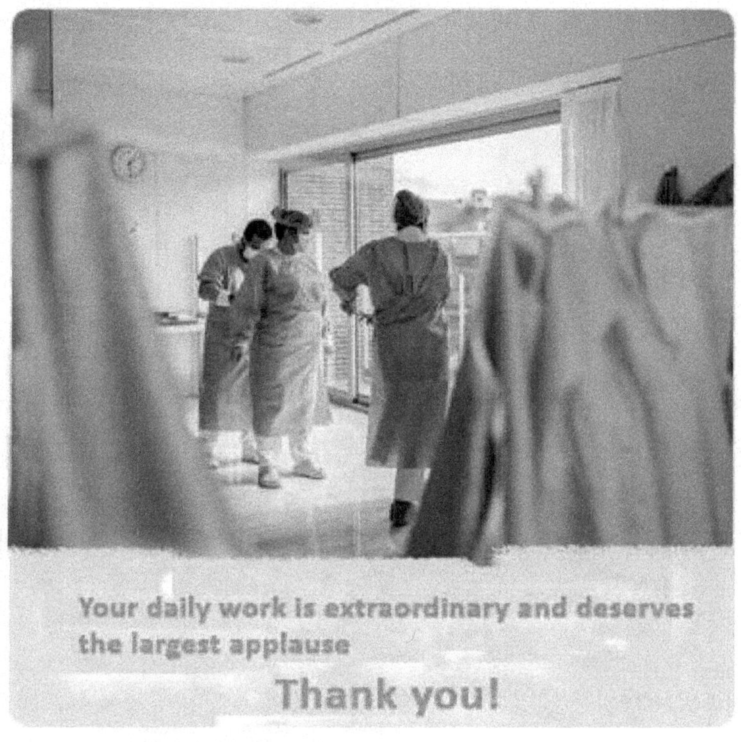

Illustration 1 Tweet Thanking Personnel

A Psychological Perspective of the Health Personnel in Times of Pandemic

Dedicated to my parents

A Psychological Perspective of the Health Personnel in
Times of Pandemic

Chapter I. Contextualizing

Before going deeper about the psychological and emotional impact of COVID-19 on Healthcare Personnel, this work must be contextualized within the framework of a pandemic that affects globally and without precedent in modern history. It has been putting in check to each one of the health systems as it has affected the population.

Despite seeing its consequences in China, where it began, sometimes, until the first cases were counted in each territory, the governments did not begin to take measures in this regard.

A chronology that has barely started a few months ago and that has been affecting more and more countries. The first cases were imported, by citizens from affected areas, who have unknowingly spread the virus around the world.

A situation in which each government have taken different measures, but in all cases, the fight for the eradication of the virus has been in charge of Health Personnel yet at risk of their own lives in the caring of patients who came requiring health care, many times, with urgency.

Healthcare in Europe

Health Personnel can be differentiated according to the category given to them in each country. For example, between medical and nursing personnel, professionals who perform complementary functions, but whose percentage of the population vary depending on the European country which is being talked about.

Thus, and in the specific case of Spain, this is above the European average in terms of the number of medical professionals working in healthcare, this average is 3.6 per 1,000 inhabitants in 2019; while in the case of nurses, Spain is below the average, whose percentage in 2019 at the European level was 8.5 per 1,000 inhabitants.

Greece, Austria and Portugal are the countries with a higher ratio of doctors in the European Union, and those with a lower ratio, Poland, Romania and England.

Regarding the nursing community, among the countries with a higher ratio per 1,000 inhabitants are Norway, Iceland and Finland, while those with the lowest ratios in the European Union are Greece, Bulgaria and Lithuania.

Thus, Spain would be in the quadrant of more doctors and fewer nurses with respect to the European average (OECD / European Observatory on Health Systems and Policies, 2019) (see Illustration 2).

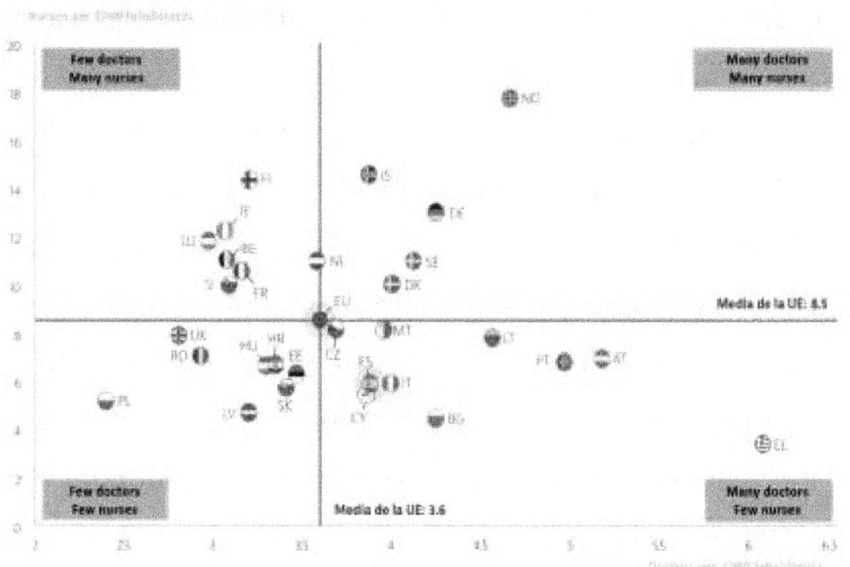

Illustration 2 Health Personnel in Europe

It is necessary to clarify, in order to offer a vision closer to reality, that in the specific case of Spain, where there is a lower ratio than the European average of nurses, that this is not due to a lack of personnel, but because there are not counted the nursing assistants, despite the fact that in other European countries they are equated in functions with nurses.

It is also reported that in the case of Greece and Portugal, the number of doctors who are licensed to practice is counted, and not so those who work in health centres, hence their percentage is above the European average.

With this first approach, it is wanted to offer a general overview of the Health Personnel that each country had, and specifically Spain, all of this prior to the appearance of COVID-19, an aspect that is relevant in terms of the human resources that are going to be fighting the advance of this disease, a panorama that, as will be explained, has changed rapidly in terms of availability and the need for new professionals.

This reflects the enormous differences between countries of the European Union, which in first place could be counting for a greater or lesser workload that the said personnel will have to bear, thus, the more doctors and nurses per 100,000 inhabitants, the easier the attention to population will be, since it will be more human resources, at least that is what could be thought before learning about some events that have changed the reality of these personnel in weeks.

But before proceeding, it is necessary to comment that there are also other indicators to take into account to know the "strength" of the health system of each country, so we can look at the number of hospital beds available, thus with data from 2014 the average of the European Union, there are 372 beds per 100,000 inhabitants, Spain being below the average with 242 beds (Eurostat, 2020) (see Illustration 3).

The countries with the highest number of available beds between 2014 and 2015 were Bulgaria, Germany and Lithuania (with 616, 601 and 557 beds per 100,000 inhabitants respectively); while those with fewer beds were Sweden, England and Spain (with 203, 211 and 242 beds per 100,000 inhabitants respectively)

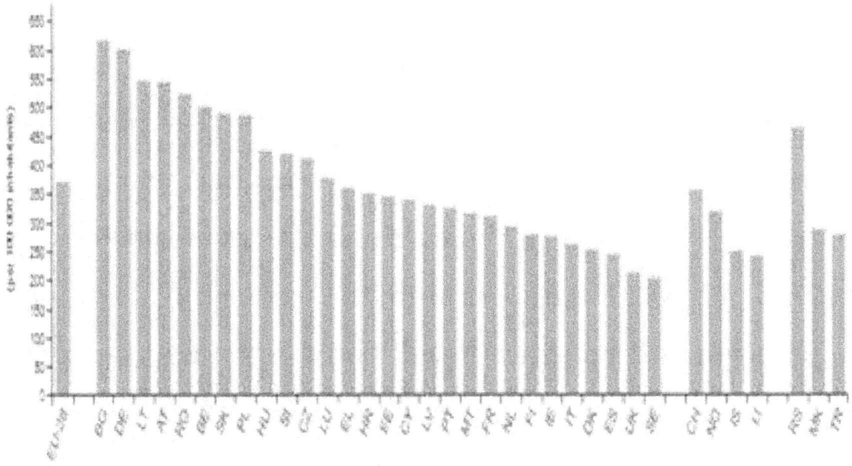

Illustration 3: Beds available per 100,000 inhabitants

Therefore, and based on the previous data, it can be said that the countries of the European Union that have more personnel and material resources to face better a health crisis would be Greece, Austria and Portugal in number of doctors; Norway, Iceland and Finland in number of nurses; and Bulgaria, Germany and Lithuania in number of hospital beds.

And on the contrary, those who are "worst" prepared to face a health crisis would be Poland, Romania and England in number of doctors; Greece, Bulgaria and Lithuania in number of nurses; and Sweden, England and Spain in number of beds available.

In the specific case of Spain, with respect to the average of the European Union, there would be more doctors than the average and fewer nurses, taking into account the caveat indicating that auxiliary personnel who also perform their role in Health Centres are not included in this account (OECD / European Observatory on Health Systems and Policies, 2019).

Regarding the criterion of available beds per 100,000 inhabitants, as of 2015, Spain was below the average in particular with 43% fewer beds available per 100,000 inhabitants (O.M.S., 2020a).

Although the foregoing does not allow us to establish distinctions in terms of efficiency criteria, quality of the caring offered, ease of access or the users satisfaction with the hospital service in each country and specifically in Spain, it does offer an overview of the strength or weakness depending on the material and human resources available prior to the onset of the global health crisis.

Regarding the quality of the caring, it must be taken into account that when a person is hospitalized, either for an upcoming operation or to recover from a trauma or intervention, in these cases patients usually spends days and even weeks in the hospital. In this "short" period of time, you will receive a "visit" from Healthcare Personnel, which includes the doctor who monitors the patient's progress.

While it is true that the caring can be good in the hospital, sometimes patients and relatives may complain about the "coldness" of its personnel, since they fulfil their function, but sometimes interacting as little as possible with the patient or the patient´s family members.

A situation that has been seen as unnecessary and in some cases even detrimental for the proper functioning of the hospital, where aspects of the patient's physical recovery are usually prioritized over emotional ones.

Despite this, some Health Centres work closely with clinical psychologists, who train Health Personnel to properly relate and communicate with patients.

Most of all, when "bad news" have to be given, where especially careful is needed in saying it, and it is necessary to know how to deal with the reactions from patients, which can range from a rapid decline in mood, to an outbreak of anger.

But while it is true that knowing how to communicate is important, it is not enough for a quality doctor-patient relationship, so what should be done to improve patient caring?

This is what has been tried to answer with a study carried out by the Nursing Care Research Center, the School of Nursing and Midwifery, together with the Firoozgar Hospital of the University of Medical Sciences of Iran; the Rajaie Center for Research and Cardiovascular Medicine of the University of Medical Sciences of Iran; and Tehran University of Medical Sciences (Iran) (Khaleghparast et al., 2016).

The study was a qualitative one, in which 51 hospital users were interviewed, including patients, relatives and Health Personnel.

The subject of the semi-structured interview was about the centre's medical visit policies, paying special attention to the comparison between restrictive and open policies.

A Psychological Perspective of the Health Personnel in Times of Pandemic

The former, restrictive patient care policies are governed by a pre-established visit schedule for healthcare personnel, where both the time of the visit is set, as well as the duration of the visit.

In the latter, in open patient care policies, there is no visiting schedule or restriction on the time spent with the patient.

The answers of the three groups, patients, relatives and Health Personnel were categorized in order to analyse it. Thus, on restrictive policies, the results show the advantages that avoid chaos; guarantees medical visits even to patients who do not want visits; controls infections; offers regularity and stability to the personnel; and in disadvantages; lack of emotional "connection"; lack of information about the patient's condition; and a limited professional visit time.

With respect to open policies, the results indicate the advantages of reducing stress and increasing patient safety; helps the family with the patient's primary care; provides education to patients and families; a better environment is created in the doctor-patient relationship; and in disadvantages the violation of the privacy of the patient and interference with the treatment

As the authors point out, new research is required

before any conclusions can be drawn in this regard, mainly due to the small number of study participants and the qualitative methodology used. Despite this, it should be noted that restrictive policies guarantee the doctor's visit once a day; something that is perceived as insufficient for both patients and families. Likewise, the Healthcare Personnel feels more comfortable with open policies, since without losing professionalism they can offer more personalized and quality patient caring.

Despite the advantages of one system or the other, it must be taken into account that the application of these results to a health center will depend a lot on its size, thus open policies seem more suitable for a health center of size medium or small; where staff can have "quality time" with their patients, without the need to adhere to a strict schedule, while in larger centres, where the number of patients per doctor is high, the best system would be that of restrictive policies, where a minimum of care is guaranteed to all patients.

Despite this, the demand from both patients and their families that Healthcare Personnel should not lose the "warmth" of human relationships during their visits, whether restrictive or open, has to be highlighted.

That is to say, and regaining the idea of this section, what has been presented is the data regarding the human

A Psychological Perspective of the Health Personnel in Times of Pandemic

resources of Health Personnel, doctors and nurses, as well as the material resources considered these as the number of beds available, not attending to other characteristics in terms of quality of the caring or how modern the technological equipment is.

To know these aspects, Health Consumer Powerhouse Ltd must be consulted which publishes the Euro Health Consumer Index annually, where 46 indicators are taken into account, including areas such as the patient´s rights or the information received, establishing from this a ranking of health systems in Europe, with Switzerland, the Netherlands and Norway having the best scores in 2018; and the worst Albania, Romania and Hungary (Health Consumer Powerhouse Ltd, 2018) (see Figure 4).

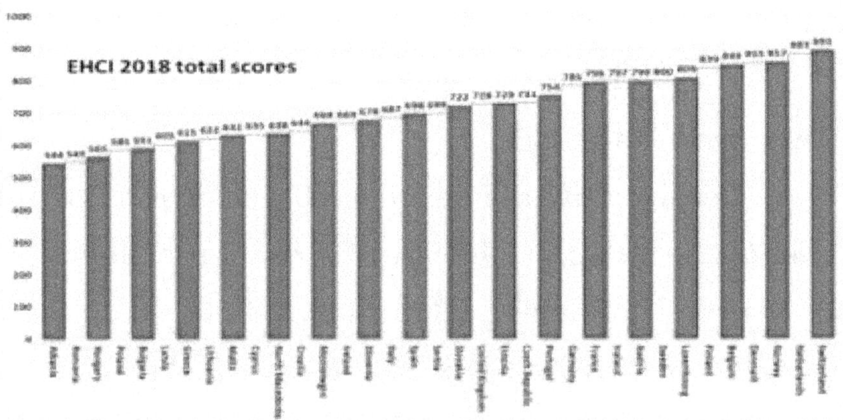

Illustration 4 European Health System Ranking

Even with all the data presented, it is not possible to establish a priori which country will better withstand a health crisis, since in these circumstances the available resources in terms of personnel and number of beds may have a greater relevance, compared with the results regarding satisfaction with the rights of the patient or information that he receives.

In addition, and alongside with the above, it must be taken into account that governments are implementing a series of measures that make the number of patients attended wherever they reach health services staggered or not, so that a "controlled" progress of a disease can be adequately cared of, by a health system with "adjusted" resources, while a "peak" of contagion and therefore of patients requiring hospitalization can cause the collapse of any health system, no matter how prepared it is.

A Psychological Perspective of the Health Personnel in
Times of Pandemic

About COVID-19

Although it is a new virus, a lot is already known
about COVID-19, starting with the family it belongs and
the characteristics of this Coronavirus (@CSIC, 2020) (see
Illustration 5)

Information has been discovered thanks to the
involvement of numerous research laboratories and
universities around the world, and having in addition for
the first time the genetic sequence of the virus released by
China as a way to stimulate the search for a cure.

These two factors have allowed that different tests
are currently being carried out throughout the world,
trying to know how to combat its advance and especially to
reduce the death rate.

From the O.M.S. answers are offered about what
COVID-19 is, what its symptoms are, how it spreads, or
what is the recovery and death rate among those infected,
and others (O.M.S., 2020b).

But despite this, various aspects are still being
investigated today for which there is still no answer,
especially in relation to an effective treatment, both
preventive and to reduce the consequences of the disease.

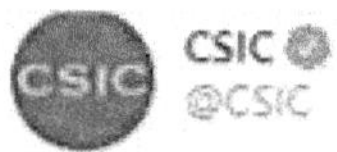

El nuevo #coronavirus se llama SARS-CoV-2 y la enfermedad que causa es la COVID-19 (Coronavirus Disease 2019).

En la imagen, virus de la familia Coronaviridae, a la que pertenece el nuevo coronavirus. (Foto tomada por el virólogo Luis Enjuanes (@CNB_CSIC)

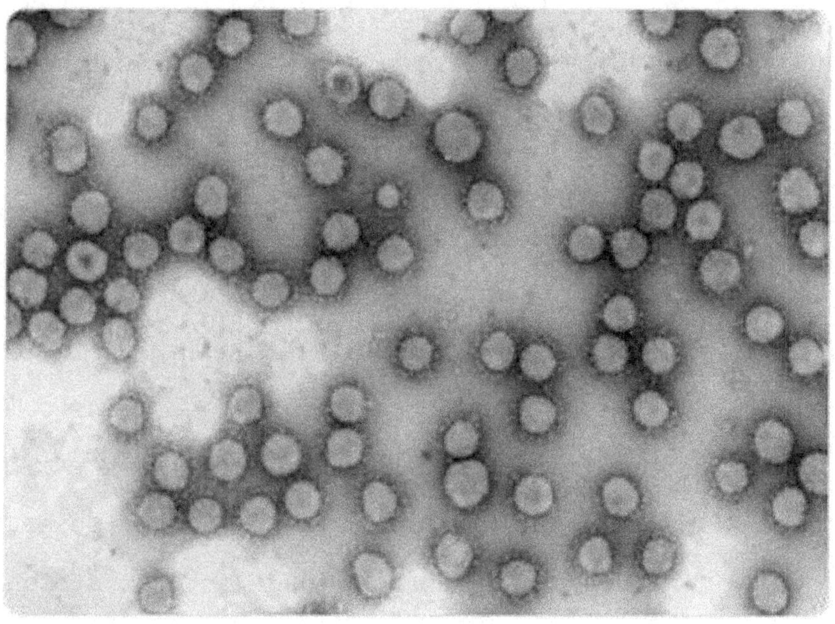

Illustration 5. Tweet Image of COVID.19

A Psychological Perspective of the Health Personnel in Times of Pandemic

The name of COVID-19

One of the problems of social psychologists is to achieve customer loyalty to a brand, this being the one we use to identify a certain person, product or company.

Normally when we think of a company like Coca-Cola, McDonald or Ikea, we usually do it with respect to the products they sell. If we look at other brands such as U.P.S., Iberia or Microsoft, we do it on the services they offer.

Something that will decisively influence the acquisition of the product or service in question, not only based on our own criteria, but also on the influence of the opinion of others and the media through advertising.

Likewise, when we think of Stephen Hawking, Barack Obama or Rafael Nadal, we no longer do so in products or services, if not because of their Personal Branding or personal brand that they have developed thanks to their scientific, political or sports careers respectively, that is, emotional aspects are associated with the brand, which can be linked to a person, company and even location.

Well, the same happens when "misfortunes" are to be called, as happens when designating tropical cyclones that annually hit a large part of the Caribbean and North America.

As reported by the World Meteorological Organization (World Meteorological Organization, 2020), these names follow pre-established lists that rotate, leaving in many the memory of the effects of Hurricane Katrina in 2005 or Ike in 2008.

Therefore, in principle, these names are not related to the date on which it occurs, the violence or the areas most affected, among these there are English or Spanish (for example, Barry or Gonzalo respectively), male or female (for example , Lorenzo or Laura respectively), but does the name of tropical cyclones have an impact on the population?

This is what has been trying to find with an investigation carried out by the Department of Administration and Companies; in conjunction with the Department of Psychology, the Communications Research Institute, and the Women and Gender Surveys Research Laboratory of the University of Illinois; together with the Department of Statistics of the Arizona State University (USA) (Jung, Shavitt, Viswanathan, & Hilbe, 2014).

The study analysed the climatic consequences of hurricanes in the United States during the last six decades, differentiating them based on masculine and feminine names, first finding that those with feminine names had been the ones that had led to the greatest destructive effects and deaths.

It must be remembered that the list of names is predetermined and that their assignment is consecutive, so a priori there is no relationship between the gender of the name and its violence, so the most surprising thing about the study is that they passed a list of names of hurricanes, 5 male and 5 female to 346 participants, so that they assessed through a Likert-type scale from 1 to 7 to what extent each of the hurricanes on the list was considered violent.

The results show that hurricanes with male names tended to be valued as more destructive than those with female names, regardless of the gender of the participants.

Which allowed us to understand why sometimes when faced with notices from the authorities, more or less attention is usually paid to prevention, for example, simply because the assigned name is male or female.

On the other hand, the name of diseases in the health field is usually indicated by acronyms that are related to some identifying characteristic of the site, symptoms or consequences.

Thus, and within the family of coronaviruses, there

have been several outbreaks before, such as in the case of SARS-CoV that emerged in China in 2002, whose initials correspond to the Severe Acute Respiratory Syndrome Coronavirus and which refers to its symptoms; the MERS-CoV that arose in Saudi Arabia in 2012 and whose initials in English refer to the Middle East Respiratory Syndrome Coronavirus, where the symptoms and location are described; and the COVID-19 that emerged in 2019 in China whose initials in English refer to the Coronavirus Disease of 2019, without making any indication of the symptoms or the town where it arose.

It should be taken in mind that the term COVID-19 has not been the first to be used for this disease but rather it has been a change introduced almost two months after the first case reported to the WHO emerged, which has led to some proposing that the motivations for modifying it by incorporating an "official" name could have been carried out to avoid the negative economic consequences of associating a type of disease with a region or population (@radioyskl, 2020) (see Illustration 6).

In this way, the aim would be to eliminate the names of "China virus" or "Wuhan virus", terms that point directly to the source of the infection.

A deference to China that some health professionals denounce, for not having the same consideration with other populations as in the case of the Middle East Respiratory Syndrome Coronavirus.

Despite the fact that an official name of COVID-19 has been given, the population has continued to use the denomination of Viruses and especially Coronavirus to learn about the symptoms, prevention measures or extension of the disease, and although it is still too early to understand the reason why the official name has "failed".

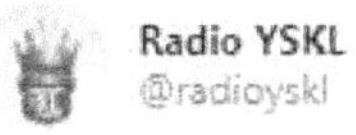

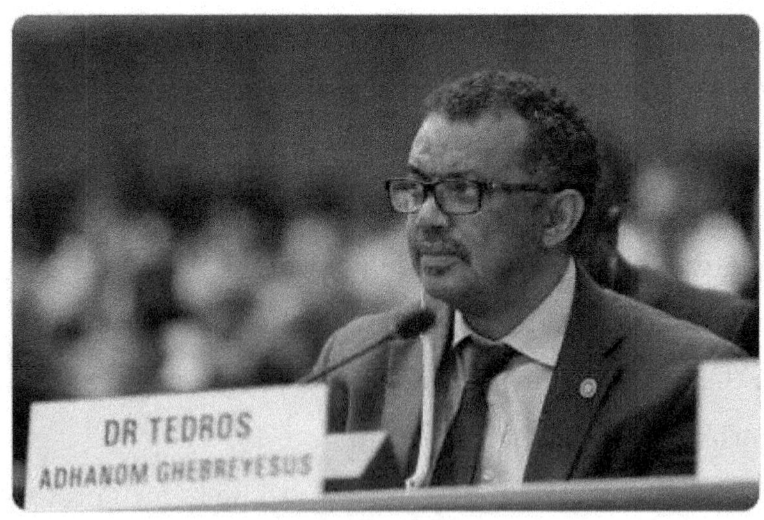

Illustration 6. Tweet Name of COVID-19

It must be taken into account that in order to create a new brand and get adherence to it, a series of variables must be addressed, as has been analysed by the University of Taylor (Malaysia) (Poon, 2016) with an investigation where an attempt has been made to find out the motivations for the success of certain brands compared to the rest, for this purpose, a list of fifty best-selling products for daily use was selected, from the two main marketing companies, to verify the effects of the brand.

After analysing the messages, pamphlets and advertising that are disseminated about these two brands by the media and the networks, it was found through the application of textual analysis and the interpretive method, that these brands were based on two pillars to maintain the loyalty of its customers.

The first one is the ability to generate positive emotions; and the second was that of the aesthetics of honesty, that is, it appears that the product actually serves what it indicates, maintaining the advertised quality standards.

Regarding the credibility of the WHO, indicate that according to the survey carried out by WIN / Gallup International (UN, 2014), this organization together with UNICEF are the highest valued international agencies worldwide, showing how 72% of those interviewed had good opinion of these organisms.

Therefore, it would be expected that citizens will gradually adopt this last name, taking into account the delay that occurred between the announcements of its official name made on February 11, 2020 (see

Illustration 6), while the worldwide concern began almost a month earlier, on January 20, 2020, in turn, almost a month after the first case was reported on December 31, 2019.

The evolution of the pandemic

Despite the fact that the circumstances are recent and do not allow us to analyse the information with a certain perspective, a small sequence of dates and data regarding the current pandemic is presented below, emphasizing information on health personnel, first in a general way and then specifically in Spain.

Thus, it should be noted that the new coronavirus 2019 (n-CoV) as it was initially named, also known as "China virus" or "Wuhan virus" which is the name of the Chinese province where the contagion began, being its official name COVID-19 according to WHO statements on February 11, 2020.

Although the first declared case of COVID-19 was at the end of December in China, some investigations indicate that several cases had previously occurred which had not been reported to the O.M.S. Likewise, there has been criticism about the late declaration of a pandemic by this organization made on that same day, March 11, 2020, when there were already more than 1,000,000 infected in the world (@radio_angelica, 2020) (see Illustration 7).

A virus, unknown until that moment, that little by little was spreading, but of which importance it seemed only that the health personnel were aware, thus the population until they saw the measures that were being adopted by the different governments, was "calm" trusting in the bonanzas of its own health system.

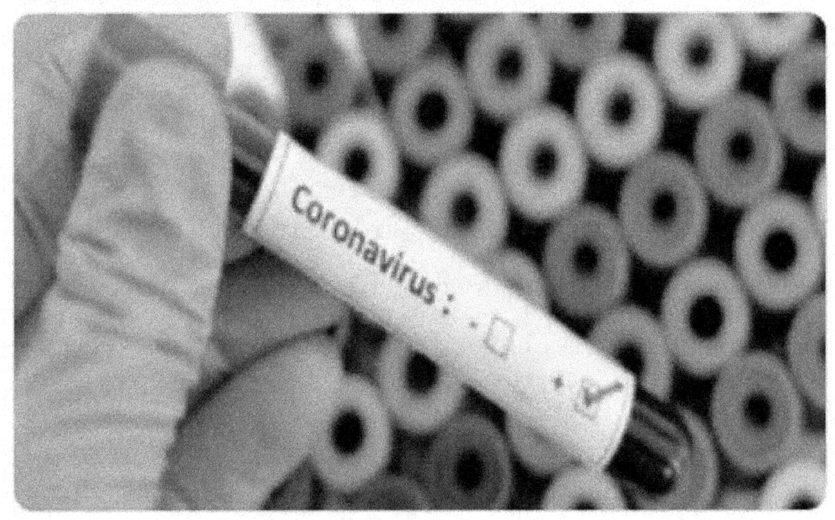

Illustration 7 Tweet Declaration of Pandemic

Perhaps the most "drastic" and unpopular measure adopted little by little by most countries as people infected with the virus were detected among their citizens, has been that of confinement at home when required, where the person must to avoid going out into the street and to do so only in justified cases since, if not, he can be arrested and taken to prison, or receive a heavy penalty for it.

The practice of confinement began in China and to the amazement of the world, where a large part of the population of the Hubei province, where is Wuhan, the city where the outbreak occurred, was confined in their homes.

A confinement that affected millions of citizens overnight, something that until then would be thought to be impossible due to the number of people involved, a decision that was adopted on January 24, 2020 (@shildalys, 2020) (see Illustration 8).

Controversial decision regarding the limitation that it supposes with respect to individual rights of movement and even work, but that it is necessary to adopt in times of health crisis if the good of the community is considered, carried out with the purpose of stopping the spread of the disease among citizens.

Aspect not always understood by the population that is confined, hence the governments have invested millions in advertising campaigns through the media and social networks to "modify" the vision of this restrictive measure, as necessary in based on the circumstances that are being experienced at that time.

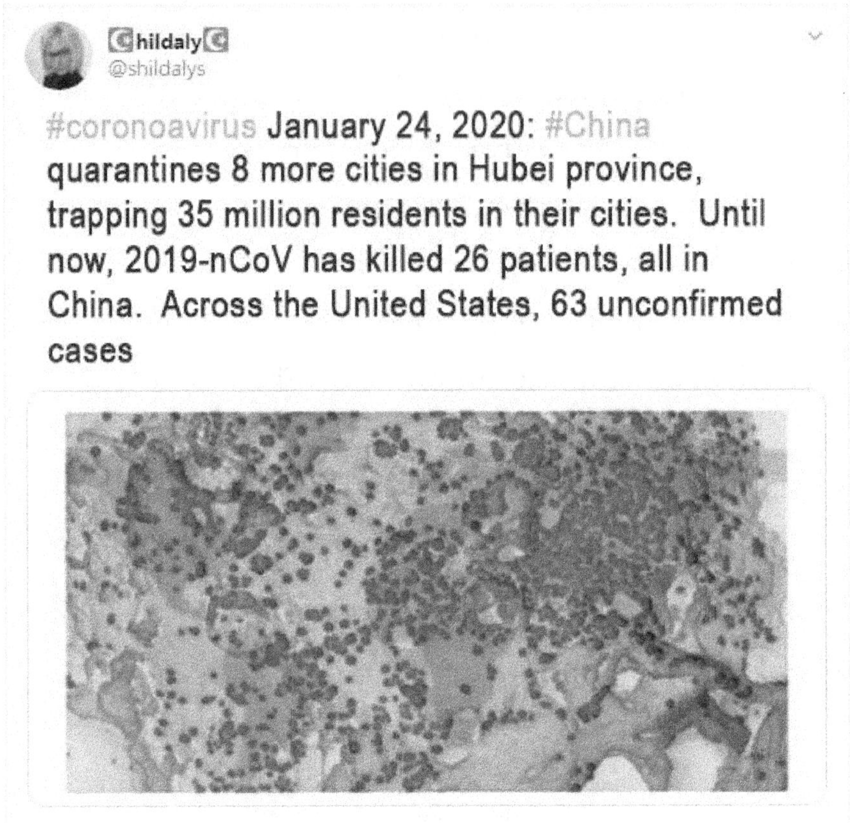

Illustration 8 Tweet about quarantine in China

After the decision taken by China and based on the growing number of cases that were beginning to be detected, Italy carried out the same restrictive measures in terms of movement in some of the northern regions, a decision adopted on the March 7, 2020, then passing the measure to the entire country, and from there to prevent the effects of the consequences of COVID-19, each country has been adopting similar measures, deciding in each case the partial or total closure of activities non-essential, or literally closing the country to prevent "infected" foreigners from bringing the disease (@Renzo_Utili, 2020) (see Illustration 9).

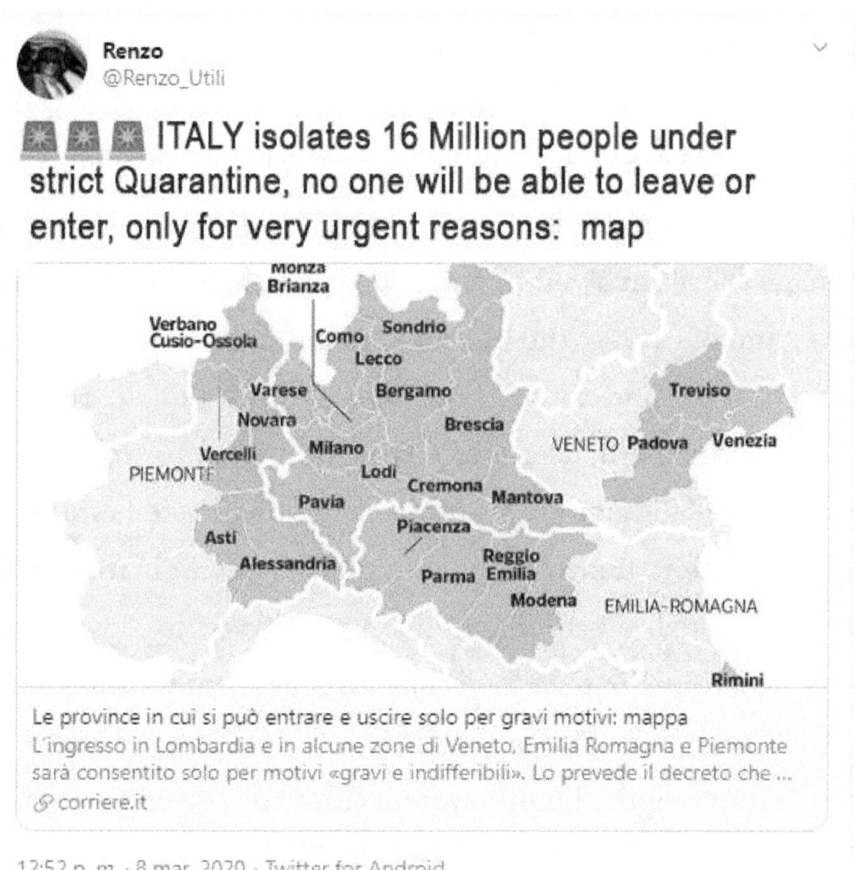

Illustration 9 Tweet about the quarantine of Italy

A Psychological Perspective of the Health Personnel in Times of Pandemic

In the specific case of Spain, the first contagion occurred on January 31, 2020, from a foreign citizen.

Situation that has required that the government have had to take measures as the number of infected and deceased has been increasing, so much so that Spain has become considered one of the main sources of contagion after China and Italy.

Being March 14 when the state of alarm was decreed and with it the confinement of the majority of the population in their homes, being exempt from this measure the essential personnel, including the bodies and security forces, those involved in the supply or the cleaning of the city, and of course, the health personnel.

They had to see how their family had to remain confined in the houses while they had to go to work daily where they did not know if they could be infected and thus expose their family to contagion. Several measures adopted, such as confinement, have served to slow down the evolution in terms of the number of new infections, which has made it possible in many localities to prevent the collapse of the health system (Instituto de Salud Carlos III, 2020) (see Illustration 10).

To exemplify this reality that is being experienced by health professionals in this fight against the consequences of COVID-19, below I transcribe an invaluable document from my point of view, since it has been the testimony of a professional who in mode of "War Report" in his own words has been collecting the day to day of how health professionals have had to deal with this pandemic.

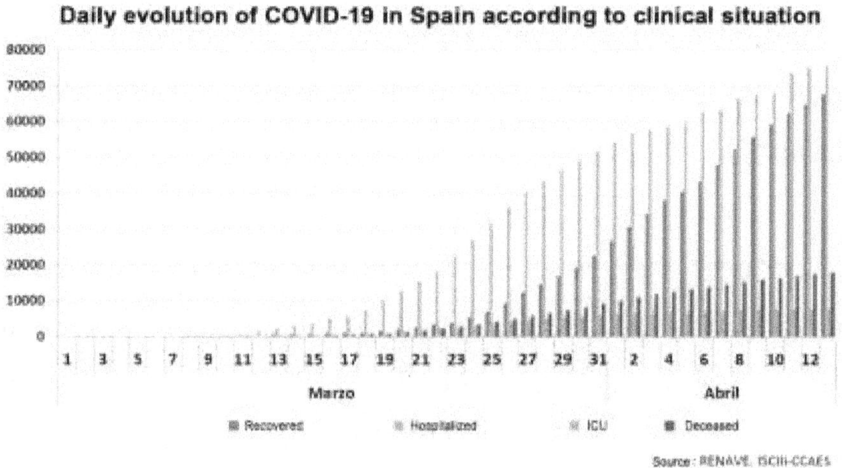

Illustration 10 Evolution of the Curve in Spain

A text written by Mr. Juan Abarca Cidon, doctor in Medicine and Surgery from the San Pablo-CEU University, currently serving as President of HM Hospitals and its CEO, in addition to being the president of the IDIS by its initials in Spanish, (Foundation (Institute for Development and Integration of Health); and the vice president of the Spanish Association of Health Law; who has also been a member of the permanent commission of the Advisory

A Psychological Perspective of the Health Personnel in
Times of Pandemic

Council of the Ministry of Health for seven years.

Thus, day by day he has been publishing and sharing this experience through social networks to make known the reality of the struggle of health professionals from a unique perspective.

A document that I share with the author's authorization and that reflects the evolution of the pandemic and its effects on both, patients and healthcare personnel.

The following publications have been extracted for their representativeness and are presented in an orderly way by dates as Dr. Juan Abarca Cidon has written them (Abarca Cidon, 2020g, 2020c, 2020j, 2020l, 2020k, 2020b, 2020m, 2020a, 2020i, 2020d, 2020h, 2020e, 2020f).

A Psychological Perspective of the Health Personnel in Times of Pandemic

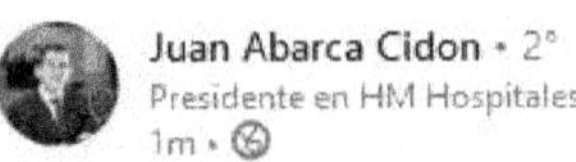

Reports of the war against the coronavirus in the HM in Madrid, March 11, 2020. Admitted 25 confirmed patients, 3 in ICU more, than 30 patients pending confirmation, dozens of emergencies with compatible symptoms. The scheduled activity of consultations and diagnostic tests begins to decrease and we begin to redistribute scheduled surgery to make room for what is to come. More than 20 isolated professionals.

There is a risk of lack of supply of certain consumable products for the protection of workers.

HM staff is amazing. The disposition and attitude. Whatever it takes. Now is when it is noticed and perceived what our profession is worth because the patient comes first and people is scared.

This has to be taken seriously and be careful with the contacts and restrictive with the measures.

We go on...

Vedi traduzione

1.098 · 61 commenti

Illustration 11 LinkedIn Report of the war against the coronavirus in HM in Madrid on March 11, 2020

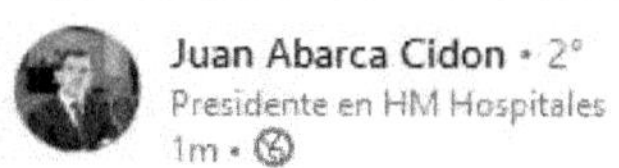

Juan Abarca Cidon · 2°
Presidente en HM Hospitales
1m · 🌐

Report of the war against coronavirus at HM hospitals on March 12. We have gone
to bed in Madrid with 38 positive cases admitted. 4 of them serious. And a few dozen
pending cases to be confirmed. Outpatient activity has dropped by half and both
we and other hospital groups have begun to reduce scheduled surgical activity and
redirect surgeries to make room for more patients (who said we prioritized money?)
We continue with worrying problems of expendable material for the protection of
the personnel that are in the process of settling with the Community of Madrid. For
true and for more than ideology. Respects to the Ministry for its coordination and
leadership on which is happening.
Yesterday we bought 15 respirators for more patients.
In other territories, public health and public services continue to be in charge, but the
pressure is beginning to be felt and it will be a matter of days that they will need us.
Here we are.
Our professionals are working hard with an admirable attitude because the most
important thing is to help our people. We are very lucky to be able to help like this.
There is no need to panic, but be cautious and follow the recommendations. It's
everything coming at once.
We go on…

Vedi traduzione

👍 😊 ❤️ 1.271 · 71 commenti

Illustration 12 LinkedIn Report of the war against coronavirus in HM

hospitals on March 12. LinkedIn

A Psychological Perspective of the Health Personnel in Times of Pandemic

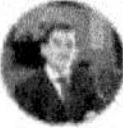

Juan Abarca Cidon · 2°
Presidente en HM Hospitales
1m ·

Good morning on Sunday March 15th. Yesterday we ended up at HM, in Madrid, with more than 80 patients admitted under insurance coverage, several very ill, and several dozen patients pending confirmation. We are still pending, that the public sector, whenever it wants to transfer patients if it needs it. 100% willing.
Outside of Madrid, the first patients begin to arrive. Just as willing for whatever it takes.
Thank you very much for your messages of support that are for our workers who, without losing their enthusiasm or smile, aware of the seriousness of the situation, follow the request of the cannon, moving between hospitals, reinforcing shifts or doing whatever is needed. So I send the message.
I believe that we are all taking the extent of what is happening and that we must take very seriously to prevent the virus from spreading further. 85% of people will not notice it, but it is very contagious and that makes "everything" come at once. We continue to adapt our facilities to accommodate the worst possible scenario. And we keep asking, we are all the same in this, that we get provided with protective equipment... that get them out from somewhere.
Thank you... we go on... this will past for sure. We have to be calm.

Vedi traduzione

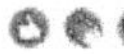

Illustration 13 LinkedIn Good morning on Sunday March 15

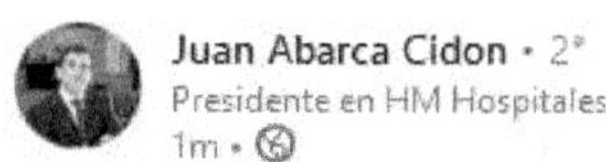

Juan Abarca Cidon · 2°
Presidente en HM Hospitales
1m · 🌐

One more day in the war against the CV at HM. Possibly, today 03/17 will be the best day of the next ones who will come because this is It complicates more and more.

Madrid yesterday 110 positives. 17 of them in the ICU and almost 60 pending confirmation. Patients began to be sent to the ICU from public centres. We are making ICU boxes in various hospitals for what is coming. All the personnel totally committed to the patients and their families. The truth is very exciting. We continue to ration the maternal protection for workers.

Outside of Madrid the movement also begins. In HM Delfos yesterday 14 suspected patients and in Galicia and Leon patients also begin to arrive. All scheduled activity has been stopped for days. But if you need something urgent on the care point, of course we are still at your disposal (https://lnkd.in/gEK2QTr). It is important not to get bad of others things please, and this will last more than 15 days...I already guarantee it.

Stay at home. It will be the only way to contain the demand, and thank you very much for your support. All of us we will come out of this much more reinforced.

Vedi traduzione

 1.186 · 89 commenti

Illustration 14 LinkedIn: Another day in the war against the CV at HM.

Possibly today 03/17

A Psychological Perspective of the Health Personnel in Times of Pandemic

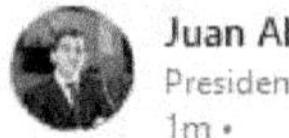

Juan Abarca Cidon · 2°
Presidente en HM Hospitales
1m ·

Good morning. We continue with our chronicles of the war against the CV at
HM Hospitals. Today is March 18 and yesterday the explosion of cases began
that we do not know how far it will take us. In Madrid yesterday we already
had more than 160 positive patients, 25 of them ill in the ICU and we have
already begun to take in patients from the Public Health. The great problem
of this epidemic, in addition to its high contagion, is that ICU patients are
admitted 2-3 weeks and at rates of 50/100/150 new ones a day, there is no
possibility of assisting them all due to the long stay they need. For our part, by
this weekend, we will have improvised 60 new ICU positions. Now we have
the problem that we lack respirators and nurses to equip them. But surely will
think of something. What we are still very scarce is protective materials for the
staff. It seems incredible but that's how we are.
HM Delfos in Barcelona and our centres in Galicia have already begun to
receive patients. In the rest of Spain they are 10 days late and I hope that
applying measures in time will be enough to not reach Madrid.
Thank you very much for your messages of support that I transfer to all the
staff who are, simply, in what is necessary to do.
Everything will be fine...

Vedi traduzione

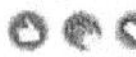 3.042 · 324 commenti

Illustration 15 LinkedIn Good morning. We continue with our chronicles of the war against the CV in HM Hospitals.

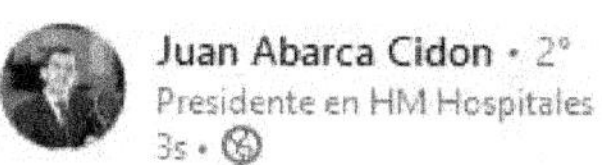

Juan Abarca Cidon · 2°
Presidente en HM Hospitales
3s ·

Report of the war against the CV on Monday 23-03
After a terrible weekend, we face Monday with concern and concern with what is to come. We are with more than 100% occupancy in Madrid with 376 patients Covid +, 52 in the ICU and 176 pending confirmation. We continue folding beds and our maintenance department manages to improvise systems to duplicate more gas installations in rooms with parts remains due to lack of supply to increase availability. We have had 26 wins yesterday and 8 casualties.
At HM Delfos we already have 60 positive patients in ICU and in the rest of the territories we remain stable.
We continue awaiting the arrival of respirators and personnel throughout the CAM. Patients who enter in a few days are already infected today and their outcome will simply depend on the means at our disposal. The more we have, the more we will save and vice versa. It would be necessary to make a count of resources at national level and make them available where they will be needed at all times. Crisis management must be centralized. Madrid and Barcelona are at the edge. Meanwhile we keep fighting with what we have. Restless. Thank you all for being there.

Vedi traduzione

2.936 · 258 commenti

Illustration 16 LinkedIn Report of the war against the CV of Monday 23-03

A Psychological Perspective of the Health Personnel in Times of Pandemic

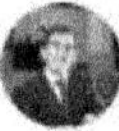

Juan Abarca Cidon · 2°
Presidente en HM Hospitales
3s · 🌐

Report of the war against the CV on March 25 at HM hospitals.

One day less. We started the hardest part of the war. Casualties are already in the hundreds but we began to add many individual victories. Yesterday in Madrid 40 victories and we have already had 19 at HM Delfos in Barcelona. We began to surround the enemy!!
In Madrid we finished yesterday with 428 positive patients, 59 in ICU and 206 pending. We have already stretched our hospitalization capacity by more than 20% and we continue to increase. We had 9 casualties yesterday.
In Barcelona 97 positive patients, 12 in the ICU and a total of 6 accumulated casualties. Galicia 13 positive patients.
We have 234 workers in isolation due to the coronavirus but we continue to find new brave men who join the battle. We have already hired more than 150 health professionals.
Days are eternal, the demonstration at the ICU is very complicated, but we continue in advance to save everyone we can. Only that matters... save as many as we can.
We began to receive reinforcements from other Autonomous Communities - all at once - and this will give us more resources to continue withstanding the force of the virus. And achieve total victory. Thank you for your messages of support, for your encouragement to continue and not faint, from home, at any time.

Vedi traduzione

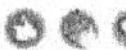 3.219 · 288 commenti

Illustration 17 LinkedIn Report of the war against the CV of March 25 in

HM Hospitals

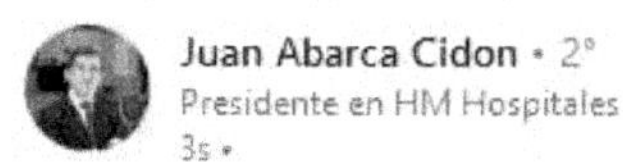

Juan Abarca Cidon · 2°
Presidente en HM Hospitales
3s ·

Report of the war against the CV on 03-27

One day less. There are many days, many battles left, but I begin to see a light in the back. Every time we know more about the behaviour of the virus and despite its force and the growth in the number of infected and sick, we are adapting and absorbing the demand from patients.
In Madrid we ended up yesterday with 578 positive patients, 76 seriously ill in the ICU. We had 55 victories and 13 casualties. In Barcelona, HM Delfos, we have 99 patients, 12 very ill in the ICU. Galicia and Leon remain contained.
I want to dedicate a few words of encouragement to the family members, in general, who have lost a loved one and, in particular, to the health workers who have suffered and continue to fight. Their pain will revert into a greater effort to destroy the virus for everyone but their effort is ... superhuman.
And those of you, who are at home, do not think that you do not help. You do it a lot being there, supporting our heroes with your messages and helping to prevent the disease from spreading with your confinement. We are one!!
The fight is fierce but we are acquiring the measure and that will lead to absolute victory. It cannot be otherwise... the virus is just evil. It supports with nothing.
We go on... until the end... without fainting...

Vedi traduzione

2.297 · 145 commenti

Illustration 18 LinkedIn Report of the war against the CV of 03/27

A Psychological Perspective of the Health Personnel in Times of Pandemic

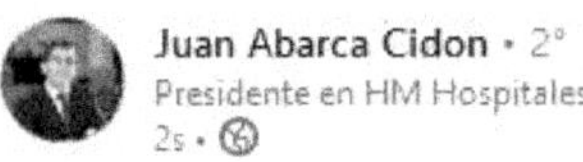

Illustration 19 LinkedIn Report of the war against the CV of HM Hospitals from 1-04

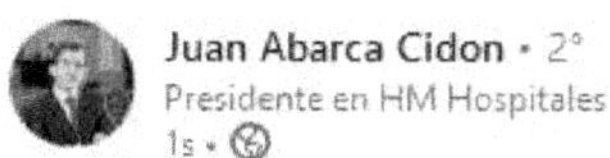

Juan Abarca Cidon · 2°
Presidente en HM Hospitales
1s ·

Report of the war against the CV on 04/07 at HM Hospitals.

We still have 2-3 weeks of very hard struggle by our health workers to save everyone we can, but because of the discipline our fellow citizens have to maintain their confinement, in the end the most important thing to stop the spread of the disease, the virus is being defeated. Despite his aggressiveness, all the planning problems and the lack of resources, we have been able to dominate it in just 4 weeks! There have been too many casualties, to none of them corresponded now. Of course, it is defeated but not dead and will return with more or less force depending on how the opening of the confinement is escalated. Now we are much more prepared, but it would not be possible to emerge unscathed from another attack of the same proportions. That is why it is essential to get that opening right. At HM Hospitals we continue with more than 100 ICU patients and we have had another 75 individual victories and fifteen casualties yesterday.
We are already close to total victory!! Victory belongs to everyone because everyone is fighting like lions, some in the vanguard and others in the rear, and this has to make us feel very proud of what we can be as a society.
We keep going! There are only a few reports left and one day less.

Vedi traduzione

Illustration 20 LinkedIn: Report of the war against the CV of 04/07 at HM Hospitals.

A Psychological Perspective of the Health Personnel in Times of Pandemic

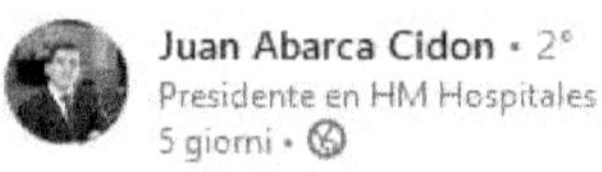

Illustration 21 LinkedIn Report of the war against the CV in HM Hospitals

from 12-04

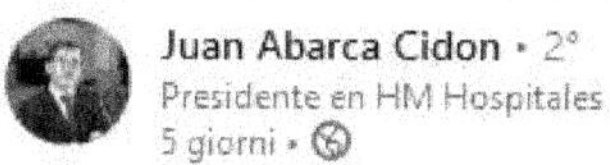

Juan Abarca Cidon · 2°
Presidente en HM Hospitales
5 giorni ·

Report of the war atHM Hospitals against the CV on 04/13

When at the beginning I spoke of war, it was because of the human and economic consequences that I believed the confrontation with the virus would have. Unfortunately this has been the case. We have won this first phase because the virus, due to the confinement, has retreated. But there have been a huge number of victims, between sick and casualties. We are entering a second phase of the war, the virus is not defeated, it is crouched and it will take advantage of any error in the planning of the opening to return with all the evil. We have to prepare.

At HM Hospitals, I hope we are wrong; we are going to prepare for the worst case scenario and save as many as we can. It is our obligation. We must acquire PPE and give the staff the break we can. I am not the one to give advice to others, but allow me 4 ideas for this phase of starting up the activity.

- Always go out with a mask. If you don't have, don't go out. That simple
- If you can telecommute, do it. Go out to the essentials.
- Avoid public transport Immunity tests guarantee that you have passed the disease but NOT that you are immune. Don't let your guard down.

We continue fighting, but now we have to plan and think.

Thank you. One day less.

Vedi traduzione

1.606 · 95 commenti

Illustration 22 LinkedIn Report of the war of HM Hospitals against the CV of 04/13

A Psychological Perspective of the Health Personnel in Times of Pandemic

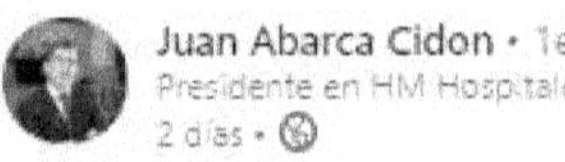

Juan Abarca Cidon · 1er
Presidente en HM Hospitales
2 días ·

Report of the war against the CV at HM Hospitals from 04-16

We are all clear about it. Objective: CV 0/0 . 0 incomes / 0 casualties. We won´t stop until we get it.
We continue one more day in this false "honeymoon". Despite the retreat of the virus, the number of daily casualties is staggering. Individual tragedies that tear entire families to the half. Let's not be fooled. Do not trust.
The healthcare pressure continues to drop and it is beginning to be detected in the staff that the situation has taken them to the limit and they collapse due to the accumulated stress. Yesterday I spoke with some who were crying, broken by exhaustion. Happy for the improvement of the situation and because the patients are less and less, they wake up and leaving out, but at the cost of tension and an effort that will cost them hard to overcome. We have set up a service for the staff with our psychologists and psychiatrists to help them recover for what may come. They have done an incredible job indeed.
At HM Hospitals we continue with about 500 admitted patients, 80 in the ICU.
At HM Delfos, in Barcelona, it was the first day that a decrease in income was really noticed. Yesterday 45 individual victories and 15 casualties. Objective: CV 0/0 . Without lowering the guard please.
One day less. Thank you very much to all.

Illustration 23 LinkedIn Report of the war against the CV at HM Hospitals from 04-16

Changes in the healthcare system

There are many changes that health care has had to face worldwide, each country implementing different measures aimed at strengthening the health system before the pandemic arrives, when they still did not have infected people, or trying to avoid the collapse of the system when they were already suffering its effects.

One of the measures that generated the greatest surprise at the beginning of the pandemic is to see how China created a hospital with a capacity for 1,000 patients out of nothing, and in just 10 days, a fact that became a milestone in health by putting on provision of the population such amount of beds.

Although each country either adopting prevention policies or due to the lack of available beds, their capacity to care for patients with a greater number of beds has been increasing in hospitals, in the case of Spain the milestone of China was exceeded, by the army personnel rising a hospital with a capacity of 5,500 patients in just 48 hours at the facilities of the Institución Ferial de Madrid (@AUGC_Comunica, 2020) (see Illustration 24 Illustration 1).

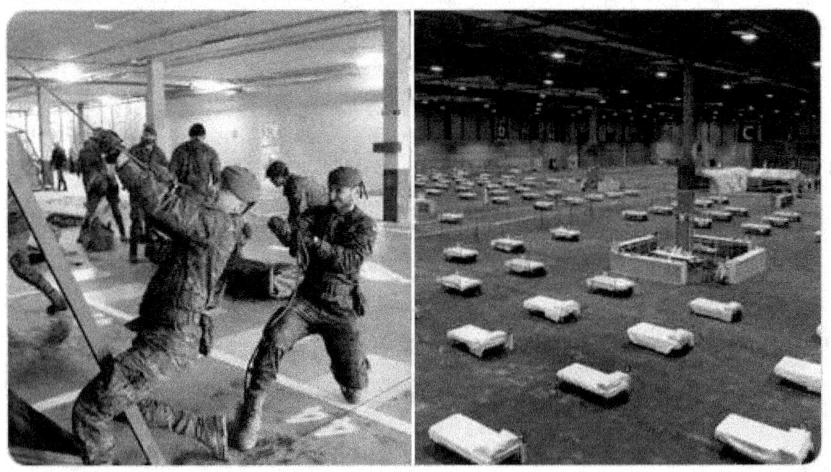

Illustration 24 Tweet about New Field Hospital

Actions such as mentioned in IFEMA have taken place on a smaller scale in different provinces as a measure to increase the capacity of hospital care and thus avoid the bankruptcy of the system that would be achieved when the number of people who required admission could not have access due to lack of beds available.

Policies and measures adopted that have caused the

aforementioned data to vary with respect to the available hospital bed resources by country, especially in Spain.

With regard to health personnel, there have been two events that have changed the numbers of doctors and nurses mentioned above, and therefore the availability of human resources when facing this pandemic, without forgetting non-health personnel who also fulfil their fundamental role.

The first milestone refers to the massive contagions that occurred and has been occurring in this population, firs, due to the ignorance that COVID-19 could be transmitted among asymptomatic patients, and secondly, due to the shortage of Personal Protective Equipment (PPE) in some centres, aspect that will be analysed below. With regard to the contagion of health personnel, in Spain it occurred when they met for example to receive some training for updating precisely on how to face this pandemic, it is so that the most qualified and updated personnel on how to face this disease has been the one that has had to be removed from their duties, to avoid spreading among their colleagues or the patients they care for.

An unprecedented situation that has led to their confinement waiting to check whether or not they present symptoms in order to be able to treat them properly, while to cover their jobs, they have had to resort to doctors and nurses from other specialties who have had to be retrained professionally to meet the new demands.

These contagions among health personnel has led the Minister of Health on March 4, 2020, in agreement with his counterparts in the autonomous communities to suspend any medical-scientific activity such as congresses, courses, workshops or conferences, to prevent professionals from becoming expose to COVID-19 (@isanidad, 2020) (see Illustration 25).

Despite this confinement by health professionals to prevent their peers from being infected, a considerable increase in cases was observed among primary care personnel, where people came looking for information or a first consultation about some symptoms that were not clearly identified, and were unknowingly exposing staff not equipped to care for asymptomatic patients, but who were infecting the virus.

Due to these cases and to prevent the number of affected among the primary care personnel from increasing, a telephone service number was enabled for the general population with which to resolve the most frequent doubts about symptoms and palliative treatments, informing the people to abstain of approaching to hospitals and health centres unless they were told to do so by phone if the seriousness of the case required it.

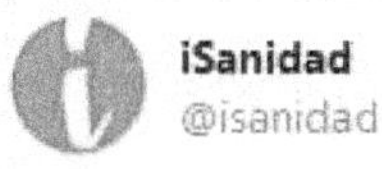

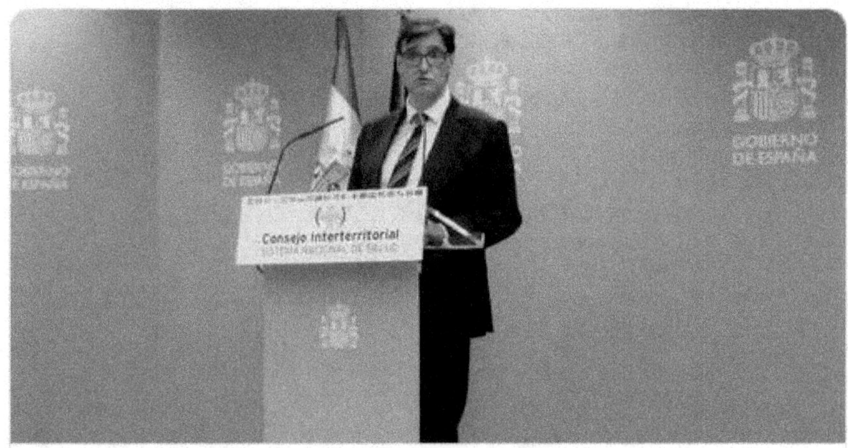

Illustration 25 Tweet Prohibition of Health Personnel Meetings

The second reason why there has been a discharge from the service and perhaps the most serious is when the personnel assigned to treat these patients in hospitals did not have the appropriate equipment to carry out their work safely.

A Psychological Perspective of the Health Personnel in
Times of Pandemic

It must be taken into account that the PPE is made up of biological protection suits, glasses, gloves, visors and masks (@JLo_RxM, 2020) (see Illustration 26).

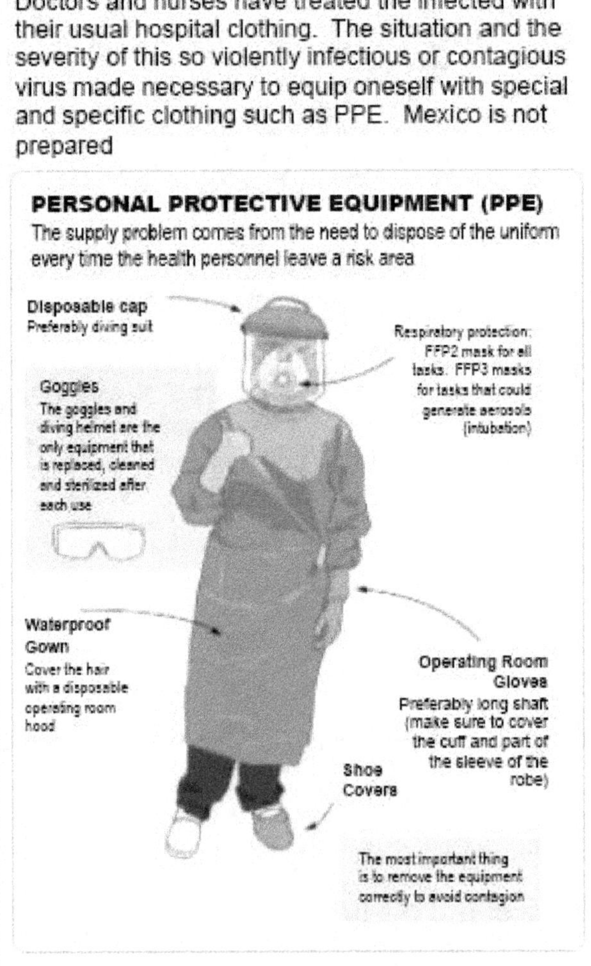

Illustration 26 Tweet PPE Healthcare Personnel

Equipment that for guaranteeing its effectiveness can only be used for a number of hours, then having to be discarded. Situation that caused the number of PPE available in hospitals and health centres to drop rapidly, having to adopt measures such as keeping PPE during longer than recommended or use non-approved equipment, a situation that has put many professionals at risk. So, paradoxically, as the number of available beds increased, the number of staff who had to care for infected patients was drastically reduced.

A situation that led various autonomous communities to take unprecedented measures, such as going to residences and specialized centres to recruit doctors to work in hospitals, and they also made public calls to reinstate retirees, and hire new personnel among those who passed and did not obtain a MIR credential, and even among those who had not finished their studies, but who were enrolled in the last course of medicine or nursing (@estrelladigital, 2020) (see Illustration 27).

Measures that have tried to compensate for the sudden and numerous loss of professionals who are confined in quarantine, without knowing at first if they are infected or not, or suffering from symptoms of COVID-19, and in the worst case, dying and in that way giving their lives to save that of others.

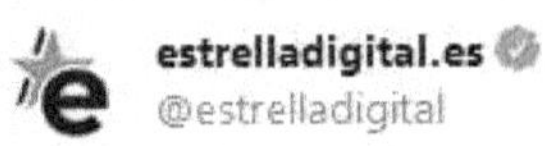

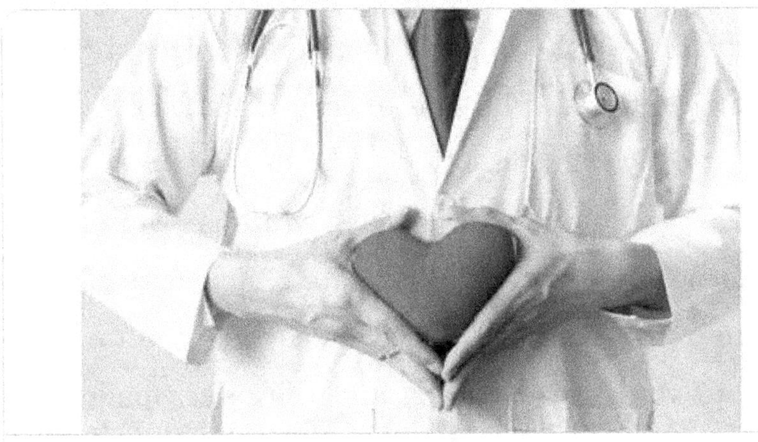

Illustration 27 Tweet Healthcare Contracts in the face of COVID-19

Therefore, indications regarding the strength or weakness of the health system based on the number of beds available, or taking into account the proportion of doctors and nurses, cannot be taken into account, since these figures have been changing in a short time, increasing in the case of available beds, and decreasing in the case of health personnel.

Chapter 2. Reaction to COVID-19

At this time, a distinction must be made between the professional and the person (father / mother, wife, brother / sister, son / daughter ...), that is, when we refer to health personnel, whether they are doctors or nurses, we must not forget that they are people performing a qualified position, but who "feel and suffer" like any other, both within their work and outside of it.

Thus, they themselves may be concerned about the possibility of getting sick, or that a relative or close friend does it, that, in addition to developing their functions in the health center, they will be aware of their loved ones, that they are well and not that they lack of anything, and if someone becomes ill, they will ensure that they are properly cared for, just as anyone does.

In addition, the concern may be greater because they know that being more exposed to the virus, they are more likely to contract it at some point, as they have seen that happens to other colleagues and in other health centres, such in Spain, as of April 11, 2020, there were already 25,000 health professionals infected by COVID-19 (@OMC_Espana, 2020a) (see Illustration 28).

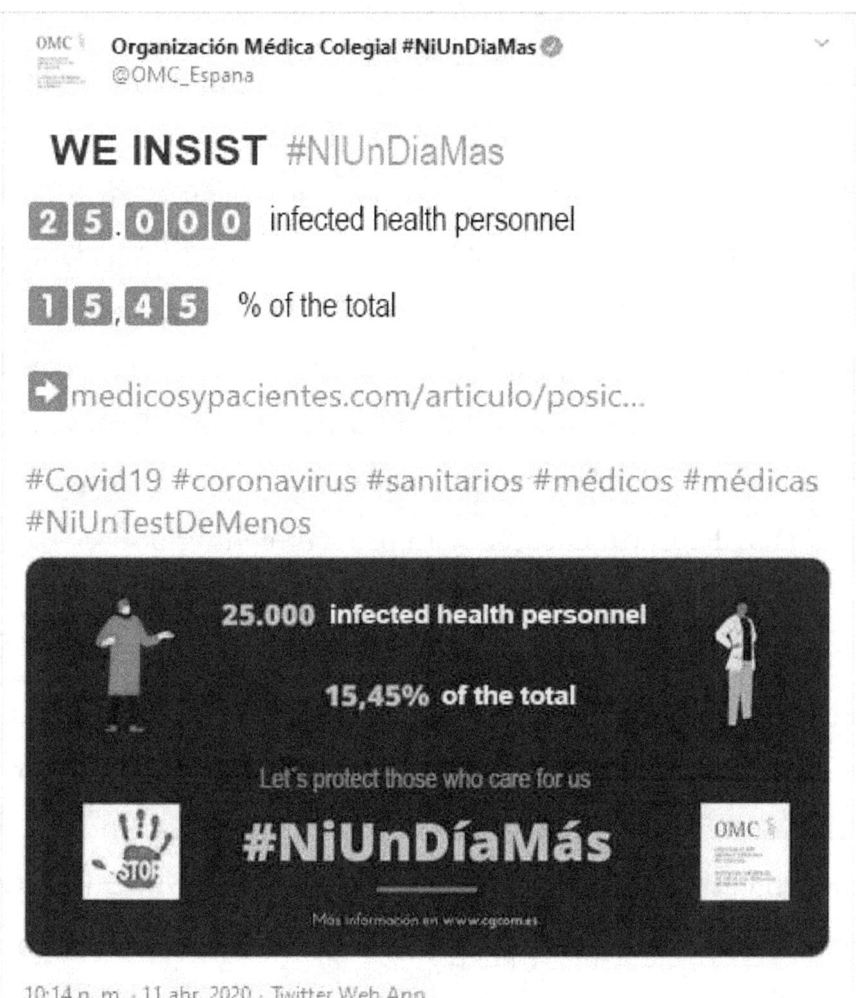

Illustration 28 Tweet Infected Healthcare Personnel

Despite the abovementioned, there are important differences in terms of the information handled by these personnel, for whom specific training is offered by professional associations, when it is not the hospitals themselves that train them to know the risks of the pandemic, thus everything related to how to do your job in the safest way possible. To this we must comment on the admonition already indicated above that some centres have been limited in terms of the availability of PPE, which has sometimes led to having to work assuming a higher risk than would correspond to them, having taken into account that they are the first front in the fight against the disease, and that PPE are necessary to prevent contagion.

It should be noted that despite the fact that COVID-19 comes from the coronavirus family and that there is already enough information about it, this particular strain was unknown in terms of its effectiveness in the infection, the contagion capacity or the effects on patients; and it has only been as the number of infected and, unfortunately, deaths has increased, that it has been learned how this specific virus works, which is useful both to seek a better treatment and for its prevention.

Despite this, progress is being made every day in terms of learning about new characteristics of this pandemic, such as the recent report where it is recounted that the corpses of those killed by COVID-19 can spread the virus to pathologists and the rest of the personnel who have contact and manipulate the body of infected patients once they have died, an aspect that until now had not been reported in the scientific literature, and that has been known precisely from the report of the death of a pathologist from the unit of forensic medicine from a hospital in Thailand, according to the authors of the note belonging to RVT Medical Center (Thailand), together with Dr. DY Pati University (India) and Hinan Medical University (China) (Sriwijitalai & Wiwanitkit, 2020).

In this note to the editor, it is recommended that the same PPE be used as when working with infected patients as a protection measure for the personnel handling the corpses.

A circumstance that despite not having been previously reported has made some countries determine the incineration of the bodies of those infected as a sanitary measure and in view of the growing number of victims meaning that in some places not have space to bury so many.

In the case where there have been burials, in some countries it has been reported that on occasions the reunion of relatives and friends has been precisely the focus of new infections and therefore the spread of the pandemic.

The explanations for this type of contagion can be diverse, taking into account that according to the customs of each country or culture, vigils are usually held with the body present, on other occasions respect is shown to the deceased by touching it; but in most cases the coffin remains closed.

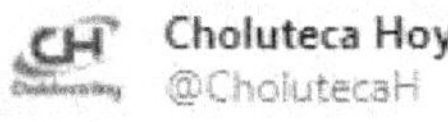

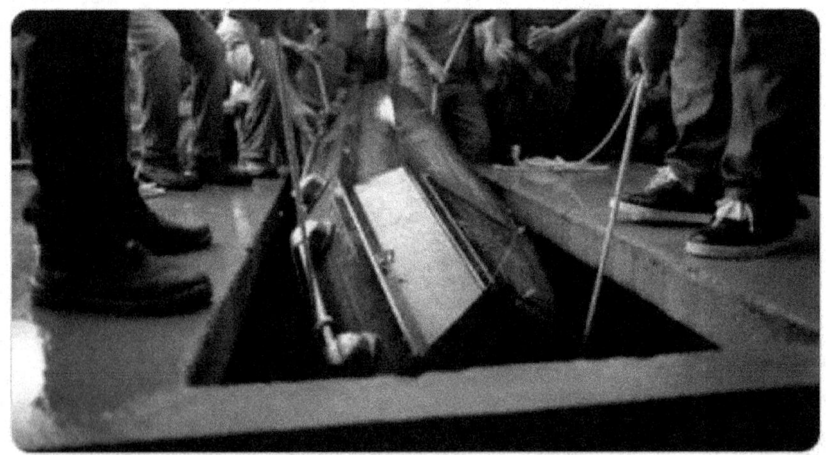

Illustration 29 Tweet Contagion at Burial

This would be a good example of the importance of knowing the latest scientific research on the new discoveries in relation to COVID-19, which, as in this case, could explain the origin of some massive infections so far reported only as an anecdotal fact but which has been repeated in various countries, with the same negative consequences on the population as the number of infected increases, which in turn return to their localities wherever they live without knowing that they are carriers, because the symptoms, if they appear, it can occur up to 15 days after infection (@CholutecaH, 2020) (see Illustration 29).

A Psychological Perspective of the Health Personnel in Times of Pandemic

Making choices

One of the big problems, when making a decision, is to know which the best alternative is. The more important the issue to be addressed or the less time you have to answer, the more "difficult" it seems to be to assume the "correct answer". Although in real life, there is no single alternative, nor will it always be entirely clear which one is more correct among the various options, so the level of anxiety generated can be so high that it can block out the person.

A prototypical case is that of students, when facing an exam, where not only the level of knowledge acquired is being evaluated, but also their self-control and their tolerance to stress.

Since a student, no matter how well prepared is, if he/she has a too high level of stress, it can block him and prevent him from performing correctly, but how does that occur?

This is what has tried to be answered with a research carried out from the Faculty of Psychology of the University of Leiden and the Institute of Brain and Cognition (Netherlands) together with the Faculty of Psychology of the German University of Sport in Cologne

(Germany) (Angelidis, Solis, Lautenbach, van der Does, & Putman, 2019), in the same participated 86 women, university students, randomly assigned in half to a group in which stress would be previously induced to a task through the Leiden Performance Anxiety Stress Procedure (Putman, Verkuil, Arias-Garcia, Pantazi, & Van Schie, 2014), leaving the rest in the control group, which did not have the social and temporal pressure that would generate additional stress to that of the test.

To check the stress levels, the Cognitive Test Anxiety Scale (Cassady & Johnson, 2002) was used; and the Spielberger's State-Trait Anxiety Inventor (Iwata et al., 1998; Spielberger, Gorsuch, & Lushene, 1970); while the Attentional Control Scale (Derryberry & Reed, 2002) was used to assess the level of attention; likewise, cardiac activity and cortisol levels in saliva were documented.

The results show that at higher levels of stress induced, worse performance in the work memory task, this interference being greater in people more sensitive to stress compared to less sensitive people.

That is, the effect of anxiety and therefore its interference in the execution of tasks depends both on an external stressor component and on the greater or lesser sensitivity to stress of the person.

Thus, and going back to the previous example, the

student who has a stress-sensitive trait, that is, who gets nervous with a little stress, will be at a disadvantage compared to his peers when it comes to responding adequately to an exam.

That is, before the same level of high external stress given by the evaluation test, the most sensitive will also experience the situation as more threatening and with it, their execution and finally, their qualification may be lower than their real learning level.

This can lead certain students, sensitive to stress, to show themselves as "bad students", not getting good grades no matter how hard they try to study, therefore, the scope of decisions, in this case in terms of responding correctly to an exam will be conditioned both by what is known, as well as by sensitivity to stress, and by the stress level of the situation itself.

In addition, it should be noted that students must learn to reduce risk behaviours, which are more frequent among adolescents, although these are not limited only to more extreme and striking behaviours such as driving at high speeds or bungee jumping; but, can risk behaviours be prevented?

This is precisely what has been investigated at the University of Oviedo (Spain) (Lana, Baizán, Faya-Ornia, &

López, 2015), with a study in which 275 nursing degree students participated.

All of them were evaluated for their level of Emotional Intelligence using the standardized Schutte Emotional Intelligence Scale (Salovey & Mayer, 1990), and the risk behaviour, understood as the consumption of tobacco, alcohol, illegal drugs, as well as the execution of unhealthy diets, whether or not they were overweight, whether they were sedentary or not, their level of sun exposure, and the practice of unprotected sex, in addition, socio-demographic and life satisfaction data were collected.

The results show that those students who had high levels of Emotional Intelligence have less behaviours of excessive alcohol consumption, not following unhealthy diets and they had safe sexual practices; and, on the contrary, those who showed lower levels of Emotional Intelligence had risk behaviours in terms of increased alcohol consumption, following unhealthy diets and unprotected sexual practices.

Not obtaining significant differences in risk behaviours of tobacco or illegal drug consumption, the level of overweight, sedentary lifestyle or the level of sun exposure depending on the level of Emotional Intelligence.

The authors point out about the benefits of having high levels of Emotional Intelligence when it comes to properly managing group pressure, the main element in behaviours such as the consumption of alcohol and other socially accepted drugs.

But going back to health personnel, one of the situations that doctors in training have to learn is to make decisions, for example, in the direction and management of the human team under their charge, which means assuming responsibility for successes and failures of the staff who collaborate with them, an aspect that is learned precisely during the years of training in their hospital practices.

It should be in mind that when a person comes to a medical consultation they literally put themselves "in the hands" of the professional, so that any mistake that this commits will have a direct impact on the health of the patient, in addition to being an unnecessary expense for the health system and a reason for legal litigation in this regard.

Furthermore, when one works in a health centre or hospital, where there are twenty or thirty health professionals working there; in these cases the possibility of error is increased.

Hence the importance of following previously established action protocols, which together with the practical experience of professionals means that these errors can sometimes be avoided without major consequences for the patient's health.

But when these occur there are two possibilities: that the professional and the rest of the area personnel learn for avoid it or that nothing happens, waiting for it not to happen again.

An inadequate diagnosis, a treatment without taking into account the patient's family history ... there are many factors that can facilitate errors at any given time, but can errors be avoided in the health sphere?

This is what has tried to be answered with an investigation proposed by the University of G. d'Annunzio together with the University of Trieste (Italy) (Cortini, Pivetti, & Cervai, 2016), in which 61 professionals from Italian public health in the area of nursing and obstetrics, aged between 31 to 68 years, of which 51 were women.

All the participants responded to a self-administered scale on the learning climate (whether or not it facilitates learning from mistakes in the company); likewise, the level of work stress was evaluated through the standardized General Health Questionnaire (Werneke, Goldberg, Yalcin, & Üstün, 2000); finally, professional practice was evaluated through self-report.

The results state that both learning from mistakes

and their subsequent application in professional practice are mediated by the level of stress of the participants, that is, despite the fact that there may be an adequate climate that facilitates learning from mistakes, this it will not be put into practice if workers are under a lot of stress, repeating mistakes over and over again despite protocol specifications.

On the other hand, if health professionals have a moderate level of stress, they are capable of learning from their mistakes, of transmitting their learning to other colleagues and in this way improving professional practice, which according to the study´s authors would suppose approximately a 10% reduction in errors if the results obtained with moderate levels versus high levels of stress are compared.

Of noticing in this study, the high positive effect on the reduction of errors in professional practice intervening in a single factor such as the stress level of the staff. It must be remembered that moderate stress will not only facilitate these learning from the mistakes made, but will also have important effects on the work environment, the quality of care offered and even on the proper health of workers; and on the contrary, high levels of stress maintained over time will not only put the health personnel's own lives at risk, but will also affect their performance.

Thus, increasing awareness by health center management about the level of stress among their employees should be a priority, in order to achieve a balance between performance and stress; so that work is done at ease and offering maximum professionalism, especially in the healthcare field.

Previous research tries to bring to the fore that despite the fact that a global crisis is currently being experienced, it is easy to "forget" that health professionals must also maintain adequate levels of stress, compensated with their eight hours of sleep, both aspects that tend to take a backseat, frequently occurring cases in which health personnel work several shifts in a row to "perform more", which will inevitably lead to greater physical and emotional wear and tear, while thereby increasing the chances to make wrong decisions.

It should be noticed that despite the fact that the study plans for health personnel are designed to cover a good part of the problems that they will have to attend to in their professional lives, this sometimes means that certain casuistry may go "unnoticed" by them.

Thus, one of the greatest efforts made by the relatives of Alzheimer's patients is to give visibility to their disease so that society becomes aware of the problem.

A sensitivity that seems to have increased in recent years, thanks to the campaigns carried out and the exponential increase in cases in society.

Although there are many factors involved in the onset of Alzheimer's, age seems to stand out from the rest; which, together with the progressive aging of the population, will lead to an increase in Alzheimer's cases not seen until now.

But if there is a group that works directly with these patients and therefore their level of awareness about this problem is decisive, it is the health personnel, but can the perception of Alzheimer's disease among these personnel be modified?

This is what has been tried to find out with a research carried out from the Institute for Successful Aging of New Jersey of the School of Osteopathic Medicine at Rowan University (USA) (Garrie, Goel, & Forsberg, 2016).

Eleven university students from the health area participated in it, for which two standardized measures were used to assess the aptitude of students towards Alzheimer's patients through the Dementia Attitudes Scale (O'Connor & McFadden, 2010) and the Interpretive Phenomenological Analysis (Smith & Shinebourne, 2012).

An evaluation was carried out before and after an intervention consisting of attending a one-hour poetry workshop, where students had to help Alzheimer's patients to write poetry about love, for which they were previously trained.

The results show significant changes towards a greater acceptance of Alzheimer's disease and patients who suffer from it by students, which shows a positive effect when having direct contact with patients.

That is, in the training stage of the future health professional, in addition to the aspects of their subject, the teaching of the regulation of their own emotional states, especially those related to stress levels, and of course to have a certain level of sensitivity about the aspects in which they are going to work.

Hence, at the time of the global health crisis, the first measure adopted by professional associations and health work centres themselves was to inform and train their workers so that they were aware of the severity of the pandemic, its symptoms and treatment.

Aspect of the training that, although at the beginning it was aimed at specialized personnel, in view of the progressive decrease in "numbers" due to them themselves being infected, it has had to be extended to other health personnel in support of the former to continue maintained caring of COVID-19 patients.

In this regard, and in relation to decision-making, perhaps the most difficult moment for healthcare personnel is when they have to face the extreme situation of having to choose between two patients, for example when available resources are limited and therefore it is not possible to save both, knowing that with it one of the two can be condemned to lose his life; a circumstance that if it occurs can emotionally "mark" the health professional, hence there are protocols and systems trying to help to make the "best" decision possible.

Thus, and in the case of the current pandemic, there are recommendations on which tests to perform are the most appropriate in patients with COVID-19 based on their age and the presence or absence of comorbidity and a history of health problems, but there are also procedures for those moments in which the demand exceeds the capacity of the health centre in terms of respirators, recommendations that are aimed at helping to decide on who to give priority to in accessing said equipment.

Thus before an old man in front of an older adult, it would be given to this second; and between an older adult and a young person, to this second; and among those who belong to the same age range, priority will be given to those who do not have a history of medical problems over those who have suffered or suffer from a serious pathology.

All this based on mathematical models that are capable of predicting the evolution of patients with COVID-19 with certain parameters, based on information from previous cases that allow better decisions regarding the optimization of resources when these are scarce, being able to assess the severity of each patient and their chances of recovery based on their own history and previous cases; but, to what extent are these predictive models effective against COVID-19?

This is what has tried to answer with a research carried out jointly by more than fifteen laboratories spread over Germany and Austria, Belgium, the Netherlands and the United Kingdom (Wynants et al., 2020).

The study carried out a systematic review of the articles published or accepted for publication in indexed scientific journals dealing with diagnostic models of patients with COVID-19, as well as to estimate the number of infected existing in the general population.

Of the total of 2,696 articles published to date, only 27 articles described up to 31 different predictive models, which were analysed.

Of these, 3 models were used to predict the number of patients who would come to hospital centres infected, thereby estimating when there could be a shortage of healthcare resources and the subsequent collapse of the health system; 18 models, given the patient's symptoms, allowed calculating the probability that he was infected by COVID-19; 13 of which used artificial intelligence; the rest allow estimating the severity, evolution or even the number of days it will take to be hospitalized.

Among the sociodemographic variables taken into account are age, gender, body temperature, signs and symptoms, such as TAC, the C-reactive protein count, lactic dehydrogenase and lymphocytes.

These models define their range of efficacy between 73 and 81% of those that allow predicting the number of patients who would come to hospital centres infected; between 81 and 88% of those that allow determining, given the symptoms, that the patient was infected with COVID-19; and between 85 and 99% of the models that predict the severity, evolution or even the number of days it will require to be hospitalized.

Among the limitations of the models, it should be noted that they have been elaborated from patient data collected in China, with the exception of one of the models that was based on their own data, that is, these models can allow with a greater or lesser degree in a lower range of accuracy to determine what will happen with patients from China, despite which it is currently being used in various countries without attending to population differences. Likewise, most of them do not include complete patient data, lacking a representative sample of the control group, where cases have been excluded without due justification.

Taking into account these limitations, the study researchers warn about the extensive use of models that are not sufficiently validated for decision-making, so inappropriate measures may be being taken, that is, if the model used by healthcare personnel is not all the reliable it should, it cannot be guaranteed that the decisions adopted are the most "correct". Returning to what has been seen so far, moderate levels of stress, information and adequate training and precision of the diagnostic and prognostic models of the evolution of the disease, will be key for the best decision-making, despite which, sometimes these are not in the hands of health personnel who directly care for patients with COVID-19, but rather it can be determined by political parties who, after carrying out a cost-benefit analysis and in order to optimize the available resources, can adopt decisions aiming to offer these scarce resources to those who are understood to have a greater chance of overcoming the disease (@moedetriana, 2020) (see Illustration 30), that is, these political decisions would be aiming to facilitate access to those infected who are physically stronger when it comes to coping with the disease, leaving for a "second moment" or without attending to those which by age are more weakened. Decisions that are justified as a preventive measure to avoid the collapse of the health system that may occur when the number of hospital beds or available equipment falls below the existing demand at any given time.

Which, unintentionally, and given the need to prioritize, can lead to unprotect certain groups, given their greater vulnerability to contagion, but above all due to higher mortality among said population, as for example in the case of the elderly.

Decisions taken by some governments, which prevents health personnel from having to face this type of approach to decide which patient is going to be treated and which is not, knowing that with this the chances of survival of the second will decrease considerably, a measure criticized by other governments for being unsupportive, considering that health protection should be for all citizens and not only for those who have a better chance of overcoming the disease, but how is it possible that these types of decisions are adopted from a public level like it is the government of a country?

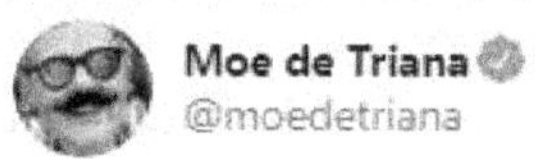

Illustration 30 Tweet Holland and COVID-19

This could be explained taking into account the results obtained by an investigation carried out jointly by the University of Cambridge (England), together with the University of Radboud and the U.M.C.   St. Radboud (Netherlands) (van den Bos, Jolles, & Homberg, 2013); in whose study an exhaustive review of published articles on decision making is carried out.

Thus, the different factors that influence when deciding between various options are analysed, paying special attention to the social influence of the context as a modulator of our own decisions, either from the learning of behaviour patterns and values given by social learning, or by phenomena such as group pressure, social conformism, cooperation and social stress among others, all modulated by the field of emotions.

The results of the study report that, compared to any other variable analysed, what will "weigh" the most when making a decision, even those that have a greater impact on citizens, for example, because they are adopted by a government, in the first place it will be "what will they say", that is to say, it is almost exclusively attended to how this measure will be received.

But while these decisions in times of crisis are aimed at improving health care among those who have the best chance of surviving the negative effects of COVID-19 infection, in the field of health there are many cases of how to work with the population so that it also participates in decision-making, especially for patients, promoting among them an altruistic purpose when the moment of death arrives, which has been able to allow another person to continue living, such is the case of donations.

There are many health professionals and associations that try to make the population aware of the need to have donors, and it is through a simple gesture such as having the donor card that acceptance of the donation can be expressed.

Depending on cultural aspects, there are greater or lesser percentages of donors among the population, showing great differences from one country to another, which indicates the greater or lesser awareness of said gesture and the future positive consequences it has on the recipient, that otherwise, it is forced to continue waiting for an upcoming intervention, knowing that each day that passes without receiving the organ that fails, his quality of life worsens, hence the importance of having new donors that increase the transplantation possibilities of these patients.

With regard to the profile of the people most willing to be organ donors, these are usually precisely the relatives of the donation recipients, since they are more aware of the need, but also of the usefulness of sharing organs once they no longer serve to us. Thus, the testimony of recipients and donors makes it easier for others to become aware of this problem, and becoming donors themselves expressed through a card, which indicates the willingness to help after life.

Despite the above, not all people can be donors, nor are all organs at any given time viable for donation, which is why health personnel must determine whether or not the donation can be made, but whether the person does not have the donation card nor has he expressed his desire or intention to be a donor in life, it is more difficult for professionals to find healthy organs that can be donated, hence great efforts are made in the media and through talks and awareness days to help people see the problem, and once they are aware of it, they can become donors, but it can be predicted if someone will make the decision to be an organ donor?

This is precisely what has been tried to find out with research carried out jointly by the University of Martin-Luther and the M.S.H. School of Medicine from Hamburg (Germany) (Hübner, Mohs, & Petersen, 2014);   78 university students between the ages of 19 and 33 participated in it, of which 37 were women.

All of them were asked about their intention to become an organ donor, and they were also given an intentions test through implicit tests, using the test called Implicit Associate Test (Egloff, Schwerdtfeger, &

Schmukle, 2005; Greenwald, McGhee, & Schwartz, 1998) where it has to be valued between two stimuli presented on the screen.

The study compared the results of the explicit answers, that is, those that were expressed out loud, with the implicit ones, evaluated by the computer. Thus, it was possible to verify how the expression of the will to be a donor corresponded to the act of obtaining the donor card, and therefore it was a better prediction than the implicit tests used.

Aspect that comes in contradiction with the results found in other areas such as advertising, where participants are interviewed and tested in different ways to find out their opinion about a new product or service, and it is usual that what they say does not always correspond with the consequence of buying or acquiring the product.

Perhaps the main difference is that when one has to face these types of decisions, it is not done lightly, but rather meditated and thinking about it, so when someone is asked, their answer is already sufficiently established in the person, which is later verified in the conduct of obtaining the donor card, as one more and natural step to the personal decision adopted in this regard.

In the study, it would be necessary to verify what

psychological mechanisms may be involved in changing of opinion, to be able to use them in the different awareness campaigns that are carried out annually and thus increase their effect, achieving a greater number of people willing to donate their organs in the end of their lives and with it, and the most important thing, to be able to give health and extend the life of other people in need of these organs.

Therefore, and returning to the issue of decisions in the field of health, this will take into account both, the medical reports and the opinion of the patients and their relatives when the situation requires it, which will mitigate the emotional consequences of said decision in the health personnel in case of patient´s death.

The greater this impact the more unforeseen the circumstance that leads to the loss of the patient, as shown by an investigation carried out from the School of Psychology and the Center for Translational Neuroscience and Mental Health of the University of Newcastle; together with the Hunter Local Health District of New England (Australia) (Ross, Sankaranarayanan, Lewin, & Hunter, 2016) where the impact on health professionals of the loss of life of a patient caused by suicide is analysed.

In the study, 135 health workers participated, aged between 21 and 64 years, of which 65.9% were women;

Among the professionals who participated were psychologists, psychiatrists, nurses, social workers and occupational therapists, who answered a questionnaire electronically about their anxiety levels through the scale called State-Trait Anxiety Inventory (Iwata et al., 1998 ; Spielberger et al., 1970), their Burnout levels through the Maslach Burnout Inventory-Human Services Survey (Azeem, 2013; Christina Maslach & Jackson, 1981) and their beliefs about suicide through an ad-hoc questionnaire.

The results indicate that 70.4% of the participants had lost a patient to suicide, and also in the field of their private life 50.4% had had an experience related to suicide; furthermore, 71.9% stated that they had never received any type of training to face suicide within their work context. Among the consequences of having experienced a suicide episode at work, the participants showed higher levels of anxiety, with a greater feeling of burnout.

As the authors of the study point out, the results indicate a clear need for specialized training among health personnel in the management of suicide situations, both in the detection of symptoms that help prevent it and in dealing with it.

A reality, that of the death of patients, for which health personnel must be prepared, because, if no training is received, or any type of subsequent palliative intervention on these personnel, the worker will feel detached from that he does, losing consciousness for his profession, experiencing high levels of anxiety at work, all this coupled with a feeling of burnout.

For knowing the incidence of burnout among the nursing population, a cross-cultural study was carried out from the Department of Medicine together with the Department of Psychology of the University of Oviedo (Spain); and the School of Nursing of the University of São Paulo, together with the School of Nursing of the Federal University of Tocantins (Brazil) (Baldonedo-Mosteiro et al., 2019); 589 health workers participated in it, aged between 20 and 64 years, of which 89.47% were women; among nurses, technicians and assistants from both Spain (52.8%) and Brazil (47.2%).

All of them were administered the Maslach Burnout Inventory - Human Services Survey (C Maslach & Jackson, 1997) to evaluate the three components of burnout, emotional exhaustion, depersonalization and professional fulfilment. The results indicate that nursing personnel in Spain show significantly higher levels of depersonalization; while the Brazilian personnel do so with respect to professional achievement.

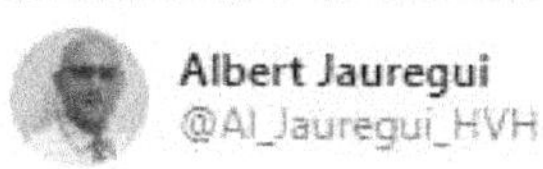

Since I was a med student, I have felt admiration for the #nursing collective. But in these days of crisis due to # COVID19 I have realized something else. Doctors cure patients, but #nursing are the ones who performs miracles @valhebron

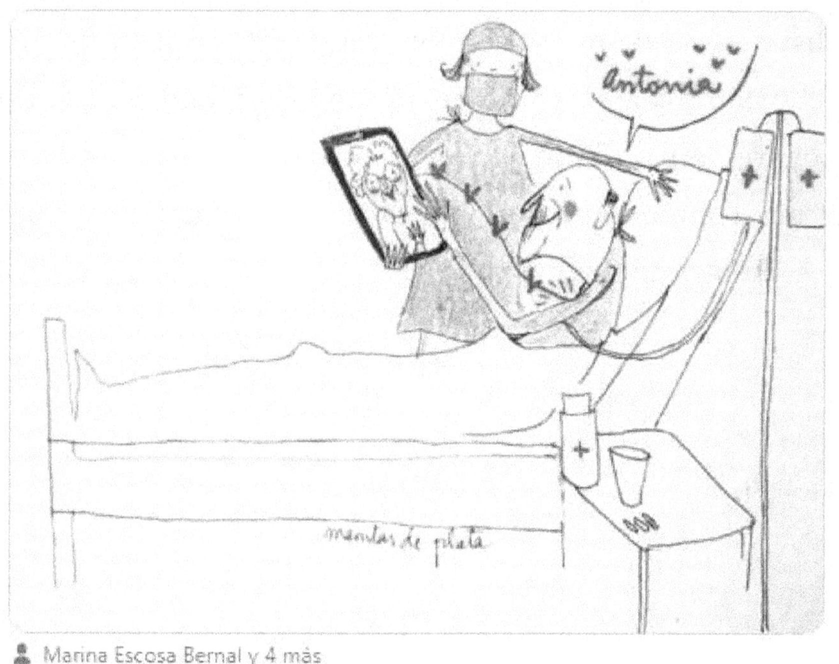

Marina Escosa Bernal y 4 más

9:44 p. m. · 16 abr. 2020 de la Vall d'Hebron, Barcelona · Twitter for iPhone

Illustration 31 Tweet Thanks to Nursing

In Spain, technical staff and nursing assistants showed significantly higher levels of emotional involvement compared to nurses.

On the other hand, in Brazil the feeling of depersonalization was greater among the nursing personnel compared to the technicians and assistants.

These differences between countries in the suffering of burnout could be explained by the economic and labour conditions, being both in Spain and in Brazil the group most exposed to suffer burnout the assistants and technicians compared to the nursing staff, and despite this they remain willing to carry out their work with the greatest humanity possible (@Al_Jauregui_HVH, 2020) (see Illustration 31).

Social phenomena

Although society is regulated by rules assumed and accepted by everyone, sometimes these rules can change the way in which individuals relate to each other, as in the case of the pandemic, where the possibilities of movement are limited for trying to stop the advancement of the disease.

A situation, that of the contagion of the population, especially among the most vulnerable sectors, has led governments to adopt unprecedented measures, as in the case of the confinement of a large part of their population.

What has forced to modify the habits of life and uses that until that moment had the citizens who have only been able to go out to supply themselves or work in some cases, but what consequences does the confinement of citizens have on psychological health?

This is what has tried to be answered with an investigation carried out from the University of Valladolid (Spain) (Odriozola-González, Planchuelo-Gómez, Irurtia-Muñiz, & Luis-García, 2020), in the study 3,550 adults participated, which responded telematically to two questionnaires, the first to assess depressive and anxiety symptoms, through the Depression Anxiety Stress Scale (Henry & Crawford, 2005); and the second to evaluate post-traumatic stress through the Impact of Event Scale (Horowitz, Wilner, & Alvarez, 1979).

The results report anxiety symptoms in 32.4% of the participants, while 37% suffered stress and 44.1% depression, with higher levels among women and young people, especially among those who showed previous problems of anxiety and depression, and who have gone through symptoms that could lead to suspect that they have had COVID-19 according to a self-report; that is, and according to these results, 1 in 3 citizens will suffer symptoms associated with emotional states, which will be mediated mainly by gender, age, and whether or not they have had a history of anxiety and depression problems prior to confinement.

Although these effects analysed are of an individual nature, society sometimes responds in unison by following a feeling of belonging, an aspect that has recently been reflected in the expression of gratitude towards the health personnel, where each someone from home usually goes out to the terrace or the window to express their support through a resounding applause, behaviour imported from the countries that have previously gone through this confinement. The intention with this small tribute is to give moral support and show that society values the effort that is being made by health personnel who are not only treating patients with COVID-19, but are exposing themselves to contagion precisely for such work.

That is to say, and as has been stated in the previous chapter, while the population remains confined to their homes with the "only" concern about how to spend their time, health personnel must go to the health centres considered by the Professionals themselves as a "war zone", where every day the life of a patient can be lost.

What has caused health personnel to be considered as "heroes" in this fight against the pandemic, hence the expressions of support and gratitude to this group have been extended, which in many cases go beyond the fulfilment of their work, exposing their own lives to save that of others, and therefore the deserved tribute with the applause, an aspect that has even extended to the European Parliament (@EPinternacional, 2020) (see Illustration 32).

A gratitude that does not only remain in this symbolic gesture, but once known about the deficiencies suffered by some health centres in relation to the availability of PPE previously commented, and the growing number of infected among health personnel, has made react to the civil society itself, which, to the extent of its possibilities, has organized itself to respond.

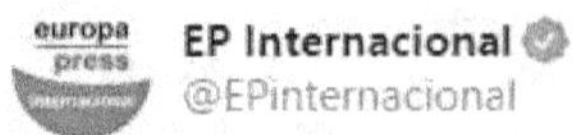

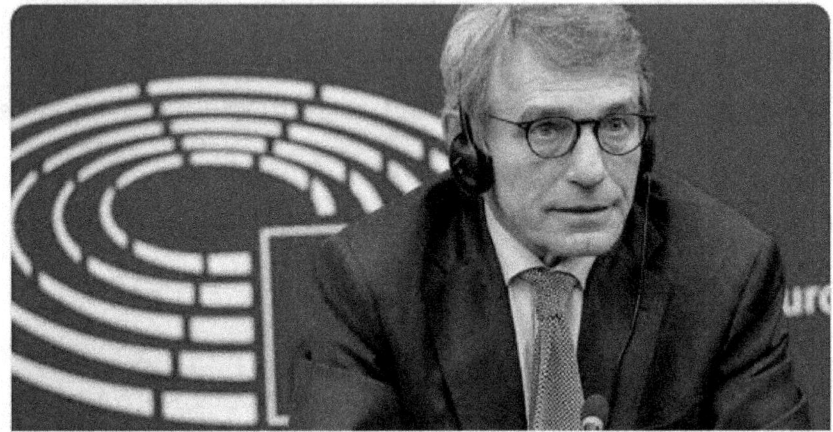

Illustration 32 Tweet Applause European Parliament

Thus, donations have been received from businessmen and anonymous people to facilitate the acquisition of this equipment for health personnel, likewise universities and research centres have made great efforts to create respirators, essentials on the treatment of patients, seeking that these be efficient and economical, with which to be able to respond to the specific demands of the centres.

And last but not least, particular initiatives have arisen to contribute from their own home, for example among users of 3D printers for printing equipment for hospitals, or even in the case of the manufacture of masks, citizens have turned to this work, with a feeling that they are really doing something now to fight the negative effects of COVID-19 (@Newtral, 2020) (see Illustration 33). Although not all the feelings expressed collectively have a positive character, thus one of the aspects most feared by the rulers is uncontrolled mass movements, since this can generate chaos and endanger the very survival of society, in this case due to the possibility of contagion of COVID-19.

Although the mass movement is an aspect of study and analysis by sociology, there is a fundamental psychological component, emotions, which are part of our life, whether we are aware of it or not, and are present in each one of the actions and decisions we make, hence the importance of their study.

Irrational behaviours on its side are based on a cognitive component where they would act differently than expected depending on the circumstances and the society in which they are found.

A Psychological Perspective of the Health Personnel in Times of Pandemic

Where the emotional "contagion" can be produced in the masses when certain beliefs that generate a feeling are spread more or less uncontrollably, whether positive or negative, being this greater insofar as it affects emotions of high activation such as euphoria, anger or rage, and above all that are related to the primary emotions, anger, joy, sadness and fear.

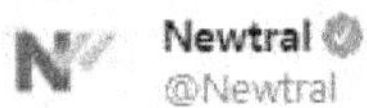

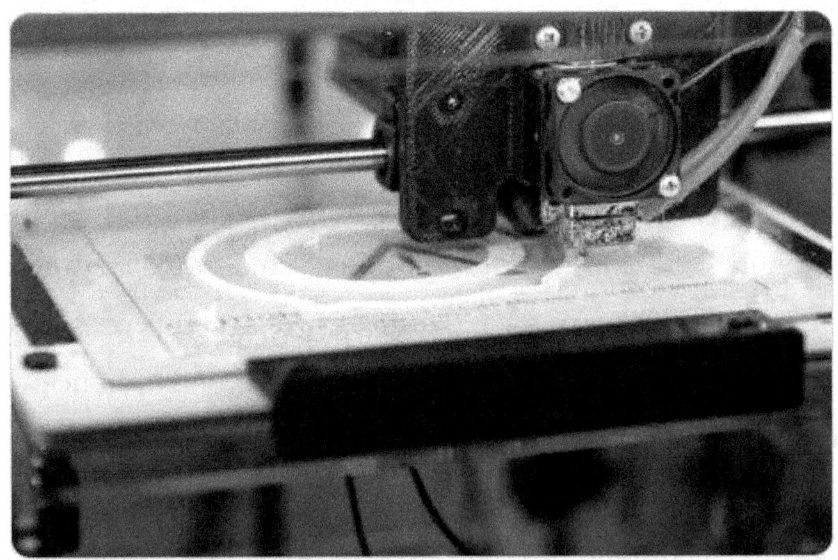

Illustration 33 Tweet 3D Printer Volunteers

It is precisely based on this last feeling of fear, which gets to be contagious in the community, given the belief of the possibility of being infected, on which the recent increase in both verbal and physical aggression in the work centres by the family.

And even and already entering the personal sphere, "pressures" have been received in writing in the form of "notes" published in public spaces such as in elevators, informing about which person who works in a health centre attending or not treating patients infected with COVID-19 are not welcome in said building where they have their home, it has also occurred that some landlords have not allowed to renew the rental contract to the health personnel, which undoubtedly aggravates the pressure that this group suffers from work, by avoiding them from having a place to rest, which has led some health workers to "live" in the workplace itself.

There have also been cases that when they went daily to their workplace, to "save lives", some citizens do not allow them access to public transport by rebuking them, and their private property of these personnel has also been damaged with graffiti offensive allusions as a way of trying to intimidate them (@FuerzasDelOrden, 2020) (see Illustration 34).

A Psychological Perspective of the Health Personnel in Times of Pandemic

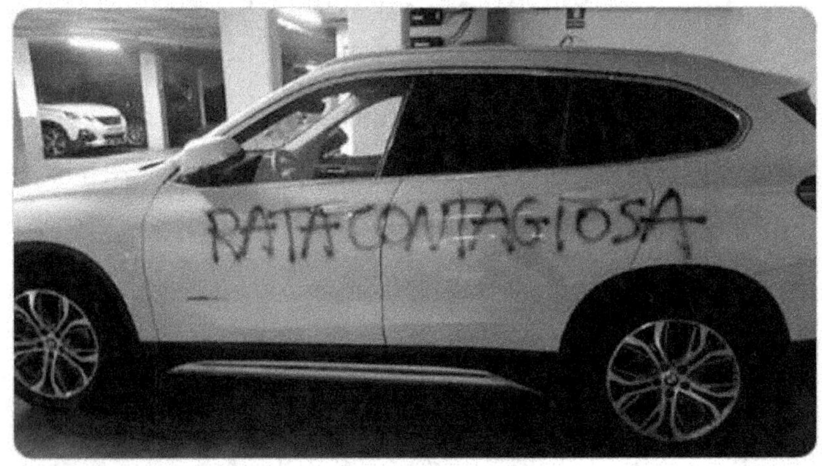

Illustration 34 Tweet Graffiti to Health Personnel

But although an exceptional situation is being experienced in the face of the pandemic, it must not be forgotten that the health community has been suffering in recent years important problems in terms of citizen contact, where the demands of professionals accumulate day by day complaining of the mistreatment received, sometimes insults, threats and even physical attacks by patients and relatives.

A situation that strangely goes unnoticed on most occasions by the media despite being a "historical" claim and that has been aggravated in recent years.

From the General Nursing Council, which offers the results of a study carried out on 1,623 nurses in Spain on the severity and frequency of the aggressions suffered, reports that only 2 out of 10 nurses report it; while 1 in 3 has been the victim or witnesses a physical attack; and 2 out of 3 verbal attacks; being the aggressor, in more than half of the cases a relative (Consejo General de Enfermería, 2019).

A situation similar to the one that the group of educators experienced until a few years ago; especially in the secondary stages, where teachers not only where confronted and attacked, but also was bragging about it by uploaded videos on the internet.

Nowadays, and despite the fact that insults and humiliations continue occurring, especially through social networks, and especially within private groups, despite this progress in terms of the defence of privacy rights are starting to protect in the face of harassment, insults or threats committed through the Internet, which is allowing "control" this proliferation of expressions. But while legislative regulations such as Organic Law 1/2015 of March 30, by which Organic Law 10/1995 of November 23 of the Criminal Code is modified, has made possible to pursue actions until then not considered as a crime, what really was a milestone, marking a before and after regarding the control of aggression towards professionals in the educational field. This has had its normative development as in the case of the Community of Madrid through Law 2/2010, of June 15, on the Authority of the Teacher; for their part, other communities, such as Andalusia, are still in the process of their corresponding legislation (Junta de Andalucía, 2019).

Among the measures adopted or envisioned, depending on the legislative moment of each community, is to consider the aggression towards the educator as an attack on public authority, just as it would be to attack a judge or the personnel of the security forces, an aspect that was previously restricted in the educational field to educational inspectors. Another measure is that the teacher's testimony is estimated with probative value and presumption of veracity, without the need to present evidence in this regard, the other party being the one who would have to demonstrate that the facts are not like those reported by the teacher.

In addition, a fine and even jail time are established in the case of physical assaults to parents or guardians; while the minor offenders will have the obligation to economically compensate the centre for the damages that they may cause to the material or its facilities.

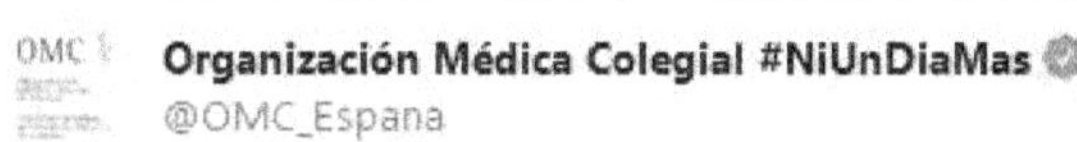

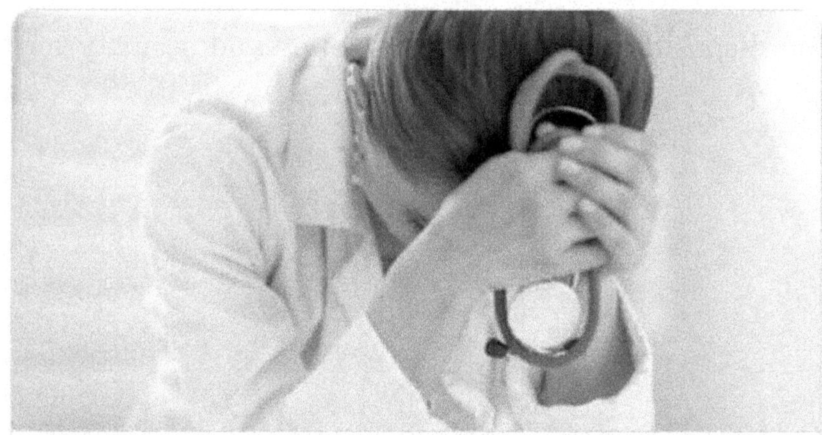

Illustration 35 Tweet Aggression Health Personnel

A Psychological Perspective of the Health Personnel in
Times of Pandemic

Undoubtedly, a great advance in terms of offering security to teachers who until then had to file a complaint with the police and present evidence to show that the attack had occurred. But in the field of health, although some progress has been made in this regard, such as the designation of March 12 as the European Day against Assaults on Healthcare Professionals for sensitizing the population about this problem, much remains to be done to provide greater protection against verbal and physical attacks, an aspect that is sometimes supplemented by the good disposition shown by the bodies and security forces (@OMC_Espana, 2020b) (see Illustration 35).

Chapter 3. Impact of COVID-19 on Healthcare Personnel

Although the confinement may be one of the most mediatic and even unpopular measures, especially when, for the first time in history, the Chinese government closed down one of its provinces, preventing the free movement of its inhabitants, and ruling that they be locked in their homes, allowing them to go out only to get food.

An unprecedented situation to the date, but which is justified by the health authorities as a way to combat the expansion of COVID-19 and thereby reduce the possibility of infecting others, a measure that to a greater or lesser degree has been adopted by many countries when the number of its infected citizens has been growing uncontrollably, from a few cases to hundreds or thousands.

A home confinement that has been preceded by the closure of educational centres and making the positions to allow it to adapt by working remotely so that economic activity was maintained as much as possible.

On the other hand, and while the majority of citizens remain at home, health personnel are called and even recruited to attend to the growing number of cases that occurred in the first days, with which is pretended to avoid the broken of the health system.

A Psychological Perspective of the Health Personnel in Times of Pandemic

But despite the fact that these personnel have not been confined and therefore have not been exposed to suffer the effects of said confinement, they are not strange to the situation, seeing how family members and friends cannot leave and in some cases they may be suffering from shortages if they have not had the opportunity to adapt to teleworking.

In other words, healthcare personnel will be subjected to a double emotional component, on the one hand, the stress of facing a situation that potentially endangers their own life by being contagious; and on the other as father / mother; son / daughter; sibling of relatives who are confined.

Situation that will affect the emotional state and mental health of these personnel, which will affect the efficiency of their work, being able to put themselves at risk of being infected by carelessness, for example, by working too tired after having worked double shifts (@Medicilio, 2020) (see Illustration 36).

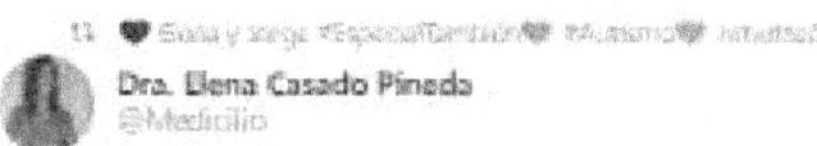

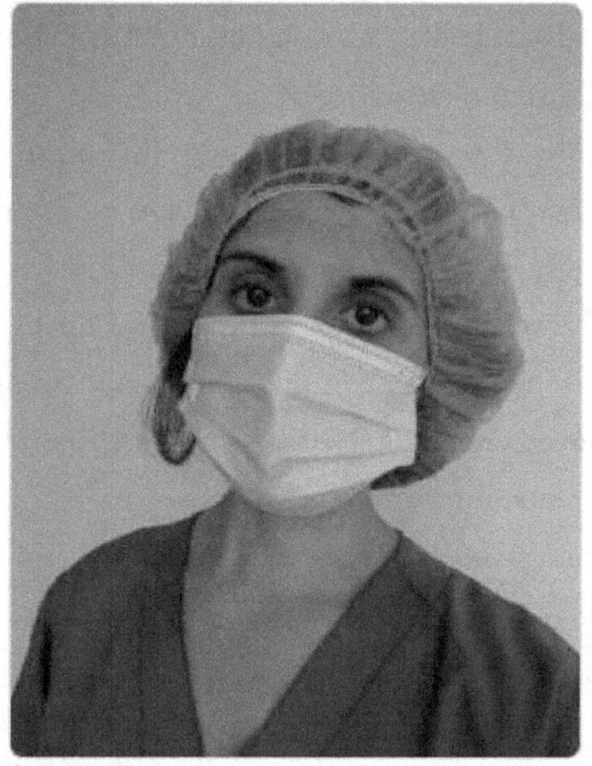

Illustration 36 Tweet Nurse Complaint

A Psychological Perspective of the Health Personnel in Times of Pandemic

Depression in Healthcare Personnel

Sadness is a state by which one stops feeling "full" or at least "normal", considered one of the basic emotions, along with happiness or fear. There are many reasons that can generate sadness, from the loss of a loved one, to not having achieved a desired goal.

Depression and based on its origin can be distinguished between exogenous and endogenous, in the first case said depression would come from external "negative" events that the person experiences and that affect their mood, for example, emotional breakdown or loss of a loved one, as the sadness caused beyond extended period of mourning.

Among the many effects of depression, it can be found that it is characterized by feelings of guilt, hopelessness and worthlessness, with negative thoughts; in addition to an increased sensitivity to pain, with persistent discomfort, digestive problems, fatigue, irritability, loss of interest in what used to be liked, difficulty to concentrate, as well as sleep disturbance, but what is the economic impact on a country of the first world of the suffering of depression among citizens?

This is precisely what has tried to be found out with

research carried out jointly by the Institute of Epidemiology, Social Medicine and Research of the Health System of the Hanover Faculty of Medicine; together with the Institute of General Practice of the Goethe University of Frankfurt; and the Institute of General Medicine and Family Medicine of the University of Friedrich-Schiller Jena (Germany) (Krauth et al., 2014).

In the study, 70 doctors from the German health system took part, who carried out a re-evaluation of their patients diagnosed with depression, at the same time that they informed them of the study and collected their consent to participate, with which in the end 626 patients completed the surveys, being 75.7% women.

Five data were collected from each participant, the medication they received, the visits to the general practitioner, the visits to the specialist, the psychotherapy they followed and the number of hospitalizations, their cost being extracted from standardized tables estimated by the Federal Statistical Office.

To verify the evolution of this expense over time, they were evaluated in three moments, the first time together with the informed consent on the reason for their participation, the second at six months and the last one a year after starting the study.

The results show that the average cost per patient

with major depression for a year is € 3,813, with no significant differences being found in healthcare spending for this pathology based on the patient's gender, despite the fact that in the study three quarters of the participants were women.

These, in macroeconomic figures, taking into account the number of patients with major depression who are cared for, generate an annual expenditure in Germany of 15.6 billion euros.

This amount seems excessive to the authors, despite being the most frequent psychological disorder among patients who come to the consultation, hence the study authors suggest carrying out greater interventions both in the early detection of this disorder and in the search for new and better techniques and therapies for reducing the number of consultations, and especially the total cost of the care received by patients with major depression.

Although the results are enlightening, they do not inform about whether it is more or less expensive than the treatment of other mental illnesses, and even other physical conditions that are treated, so it cannot be estimated if it is an excessive expense or not for administrations, or if it has to be prioritized over other diseases due to its high cost.

All of the above shows how it is not a minor problem, due to its implications both with regard to the patient and their health, as well as the economic cost it generates in the health system.

Thus, once this problem has been put into perspective, it remains to be indicated that there is a difficulty associated with this pathology, and that is that despite the fact that the health personnel itself may know about these consequences, despite this they may decide not to go to the professional of mental health to request the relevant psychological help.

There are several causes that can explain it, so it may be due to personal factors by underestimating the consequences of the emotions that are being experienced, as well as cultural factors where unlike what happens in other societies where it is seen as normal to go once to the week to the psychologist, in certain countries there is a certain suspicion about receiving professional help for emotional problems, especially when mental health is associated with social stigma in a said population.

A resistance to requesting help that can be observed among different groups of professionals, as shown by the results of an investigation carried out from Iowa State University together with Aubum University (Heath, Seidman, Vogel, Cornish, & Wade, 2017).

A Psychological Perspective of the Health Personnel in
Times of Pandemic

The study included 271 military men, aged between 24 to 38 years, 80% of whom were career professionals. All of them had to fill in the Gender Role Conflict Scale-Short Form (Wester, Vogel, O'Neil, & Danforth, 2012) to evaluate the emotions expressed; the Clinical Outcomes in Routine Evaluation (Barkham et al., 2013) to evaluate symptoms associated with stress; and the Self-Stigma of Seeking Help scale (Vogel, Wade, & Haake, 2006) to evaluate the request for psychological help.

The results report that those with high levels of anxiety and emotional restrictions come seeking psychological help; on the other hand, those who have moderate levels of anxiety and high emotional problems are significantly more reluctant to request psychological help, that is, and extrapolating these results to health personnel, they would go when they feel that their anxiety levels are high, and they not would do it when they need it most, that is, with moderate levels of anxiety but with greater emotional problems. Precisely to respond to this need for professional help from the Official Schools of Psychology, a free telephone service has been enabled for the psychological care of health personnel (@ColEnferMalaga, 2020) (see Illustration 37).

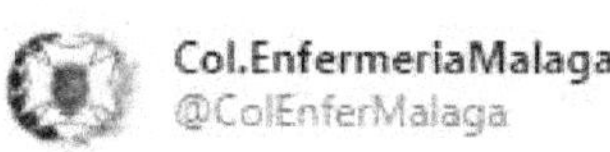

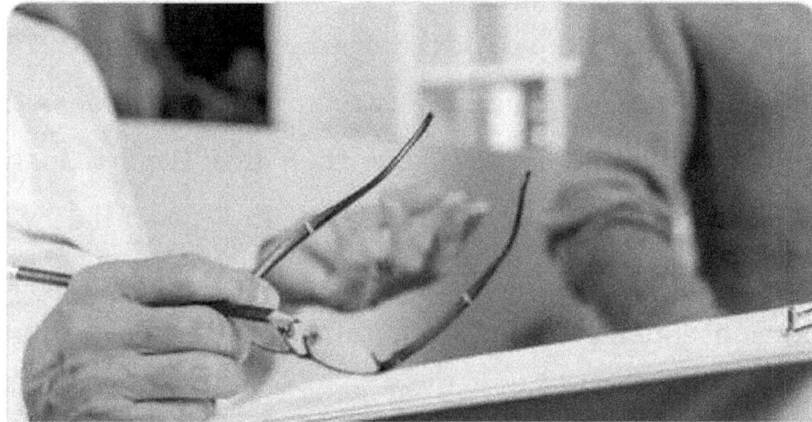

Illustration 37 Telephone for Health Personnel

Even with this availability of free help, not all health workers will be willing to call for psychological care, since despite the campaigns that are carried out annually to sensitize the population about the importance of the work of professionals of mental health there is still reluctance in society when it comes to resorting to this service, to try to understand this resistance a joint investigation has been carried out from the Australian Northern Territory Relations Agency of the Charles Darwin University together with the Federation University (Australia) (Alexi & Kathleen A. Moore, 2016).

The study compared two adult populations, the Anglo-Saxon and the Greek (with 8 and 9 participants respectively), all of them living in Australia, who underwent a semi-structured interview whose responses were subsequently categorized and analysed ,   taking into account the vision of participants on mental health and whether or not they attended a consultation.

The results show that Anglo-Saxons have fewer problems when it comes to consulting, while Greeks try to seek informal help, including religious help, to try to solve this type of problem.

Behaviour that was in accordance with the vision of mental health problems, where the Greeks showed a greater stigma in this regard, that is, seeing it as a socially rejected problem, that could make them not go to consultation, in case "someone saw them "go to that consultation.

As the authors indicate, a lot of work still needs to be done to raise awareness on population that they turn to mental health professionals when they require it, especially when in the last decade there has been a significant growth of this problem such as the WHO denounces it; hence, it is necessary for the population to have a greater awareness of what a professional on mental health is, and when to go to it.

Therefore, health professionals, in addition to attending and caring for patients, must take care of themselves, in order to avoid suffering from depressive symptoms or burnout, the latter will be characterized by fatigue, depersonalization and loss of satisfaction, which should not be confused with depressive symptoms that include depressed mood, easy crying, hopelessness, guilt, sleep disturbances, somatic symptoms, suicidal ideas, severe fatigue and irritability, but, how does each type of stress affect health?

This is what the School of Experimental Psychology at the University of Bristol (England) (Thomson, 2014) has tried to answer, for this, a study was carried out in which 1413 people participated, of which 785 had suffered depression (480 endogenous and 205 reactive), whose mean ages ranged from 44 to 58 years in which they suffered reactive depression and endogenous depression respectively, among the participants more than half, 67.7% were women. Data from the National Health Service Registry (England) were used as a control group, where information was obtained on the number of heart attacks suffered, as well as the survival rate of people with the same ages.

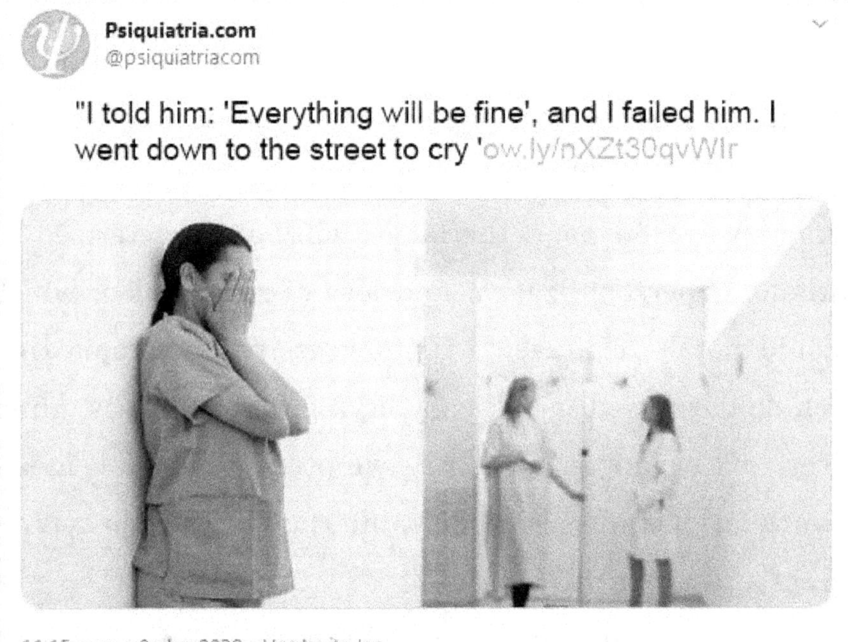

Illustration 38 Tweet Nurse Crying

The results found that men tend to suffer a significant shortening of life due to problems associated with the heart, but this relation only occurs in the case of endogenous depression; therefore, it can be concluded that depression is not a problem that should be left undiagnosed or treated within healthcare personnel since it can have important health consequences, and above all because it can shorten life if it is not received the corresponding professional help, especially when exposed to situations as serious as the death of patients (@psiquiatriacom, 2020) (see Illustration 38).

A Psychological Perspective of the Health Personnel in Times of Pandemic

Anxiety in Healthcare Personnel

Throughout the day there are numerous situations that require maximum attention, in which the best possible response has to be given, either due to haste or due to having to attend to several requirements at the same time, being that these demands can produce stress, which maintained in a medium or long term can be harmful to health, is what is known as distress, but there is also "good" stress, that is, one that for a short period of time enhances the capacities and makes give more accurate answers in the activities performed, this second type of stress is called eustress.

Whether it is "good" or "bad" depends both on the psychological assessment of stressful events and situations and on whether these remain for a certain time, thus, a situation valued as challenging, but attractive as a way to overcome or to improve, motivates to give the best of ourselves, obtaining successes that otherwise would not be achieved; but if this situation is maintained over time, the depletion of resources occurs as explained in the General Adaptation Syndrome (Selye, 1946), and with this it would cease to be motivating, becoming something "insufferable", giving success step to the   disease.   This syndrome precisely accounts for how this process is going to take place, for which it is divided into three stages:

- The initial or alarm reaction, from the moment the stimulus or stressful situation occurs, the body has to prepare to respond.

- Resistance or Adaptation, in this phase the Hypothalamic Pituitary Adrenal (H.H.A.) mechanism is set in motion to respond to the stressful demand; if this disappears, the organism will tend to a "deactivation" produced by a negative feedback mechanism, which uses the same HHA pathway, in such a way that the cortisol of the adrenal glands will inhibit the production of the corticotrophin-releasing hormone from the pituitary gland and with this will deactivate the HHA axis, thus recovering the basal levels prior to the onset of stress; on the other hand, if the stressful stimulus is maintained, the organism will go to the next phase.

- The final or exhaustion, based on the fact that the body's resources are limited and available for a short time, after which they are depleted, as well as the state of tension that originates it. This exhaustion will bring a whole series of consequences in the different systems involved that can lead the person to become ill.

Thus, a medium-term stress is going to have a series of consequences, such as muscle aches, sleep and mood disturbances and immunodeficiency; while a chronic stress on the other hand will cause more serious effects, being responsible for digestive alterations that can lead to ulcers and diarrhoea; obesity due to increased appetite and with this the possibility of suffering from diabetes increases; weakening of the immune system, being more exposed to infections and colds; loss of memory, motivation, sleep, altered mood; and increased blood pressure and heart rate, accumulation of cholesterol and triglycerides in the blood, with increased risk of heart disease and strokes.

At a psychological level, the acute toxicity of high levels of cortisol in the brain, leads to the affectation of certain neuronal structures that will affect a worse cognitive performance, as in the case of the hippocampus, necessary for the establishment of new learning; it will also increase the symptoms of certain disorders, as in the case of schizophrenia where higher levels of stress, greater expression of psychotic symptoms.

The H.H.A. therefore, will give the measure of how the body works, if it does it correctly, that is, if there is a specific activation in stressful situations, the person will be able to give the appropriate response at the moment, either escape or confrontation, while if it is maintained over time, due to the fact that the stressor is still present, "failures" will begin to occur in the normal process, and with this the probability of suffering from various diseases increases.

And this is due to the close relationship between the immune and psychological systems, since the former is essential for the correct recovery of any alteration of the organism; since low defences not only slow down this process, but also favor the appearance of infections and other diseases.

Relationship mediated by the type of personality one has, thus high levels of stress will mainly affect the health of the heart, where those who have Type A personality are especially competitive, restless and with high levels of stress and anxiety in their day to day, having a greater chance of suffering a heart disease, such as heart attack, which, if it occurs, not only increases the possibility of having another heart attack but also significantly weakens this muscle as important as the heart, being able to shorten in many cases months and even years of life. By contrast, the term type B personality emerged, as a health protector, characterized by a calm individual, with a peaceful mind, governed by values of cooperation and creativity, being able to be equally effective in their tasks; in this case, the heart, far from suffering the daily "stakes", seems to be protected and thus fewer attacks occur than in the type A personality.

But while these types of personalities are the best known, a few years ago two other types were discovered; thus, in type C personality, there is a high level of expression of emotion, particularly positive ones, with a concealment of negative emotions from other people, as a result they will be more likely to suffer rheumatism, infections, allergies, skin diseases and cancer; on the other hand, in the face of personality type D, a high level of self-demand is exhibited, with hyperactive behaviour and low self-esteem; with disconnection between the emotional world and the "rational" one, which makes them more likely to suffer psychosomatic illnesses. For all the above, it is important to avoid high levels of anxiety, knowing that depending on the type of personality it will have some effects or the others (@ 2010Asuka2010, 2020)

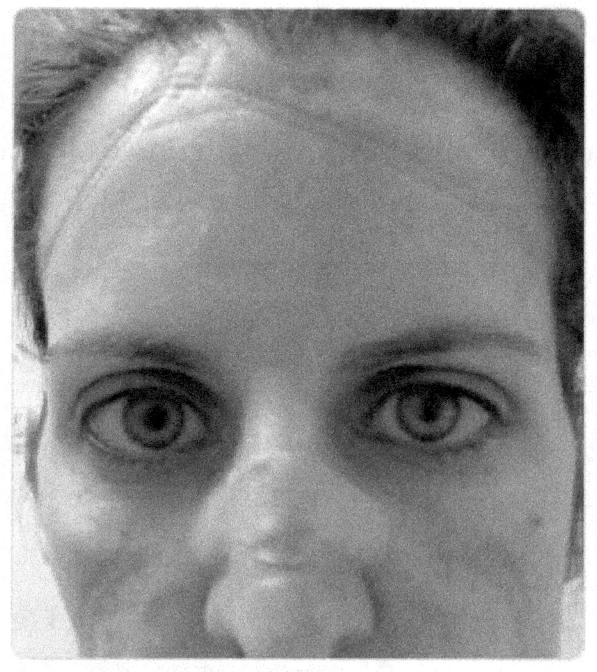

Illustration 39 Tweet Nurse Anxiety

A Psychological Perspective of the Health Personnel in Times of Pandemic

It is known that, once childhood is over, when there are greater numbers of hours of sleep than of wakefulness, the body reverses that proportion, needing around 8 hours of sleep a day for the rest of its life.

Although sometimes the administration of time is not continuous, being able to produce losses and accumulations of sleep during a time, for example, in the "shifts" of health personnel, or when continuous shifts are carried out, which recover that loss of hours of sleep that "accumulates" with a compensation of a long sleep.

But in case that sleep does not get to be recovered, the effects that its loss causes will be increasingly serious and important, affecting both physical and psychological health and social relationships; thus, it will be suffered muscle exhaustion, a greater tendency to suffer from diseases, since the immune system becomes over-activated during sleep, in addition to the injuries that lack of attention can cause, increasing the possibility of accidents; likewise, on a psychological level, there will be a reduction in the capacity for attention and concentration, with the appearance of scattered and superficial thinking.

With regard to social relationships, others will

realize this lack of sleep, and the physical and psychological consequences that it entails, and based on that they will react, to which it must be added that behaviours of not-wanting to share time with others due to excess fatigue or irascibility when interacting with others, which will lead to the loss of social contact.

The classic experiments on sleep deprivation show the devastating effects on attention, performance and other cognitive functions such as learning, even being able to put the mental health of the person at risk, which after days without sleep is tired, exhausted, but also irritable, with moments of euphoria, with paranoid thoughts, being able to suffer psychotic episodes, and all this due to not sleeping well.

Likewise, sleep deprivation will have an important effect on decision-making, according to the study carried out by the Sleep Research Center of the University of Loughborough (England) (Horne, 2012).

This has been evidenced by experiments regarding decision-making on future earnings, such as with the technique called Iowa Gambling Task (Buelow & Suhr, 2009) with which the precision in the decisions adopted can be appreciated, depending on the variables set by the experimenter, who manipulates the amount of gains or losses that can be made in each trial.

A Psychological Perspective of the Health Personnel in
Times of Pandemic

There are four possible trials depending on the established result, high gain, small gain, small loss or great loss.

Once a baseline is obtained on their performance, this method is administered after a few hours of deprivation, usually over 24 hours without sleep, to observe the interference or not of lack of sleep in the adoption of a decision, showing how errors are produced in decision making when comparing between costs and benefits, all associated with lack of sleep.

There is research like that carried out by the Division of Neuropsychiatry of the Walter Reed Armed Research Institute; the Maryland Center for Psychiatric Studies; the Department of Psychiatry at the University of Maryland; the Department of Radiology of the School of Medicine, and the Department of Environmental Health Sciences of the School of Public Health and Hygiene of the Johns Hopkins Institute of Medicine (USA) together with the Rotman Research Institute and the University of Toronto (Canada) (Colten & Altevogt, 2006) that indicate that a deprivation of 49 hours causes the participants to go for decisions where they run too much risk, as would a person injured in the ventral prefrontal cortex.

That is, lack of sleep will not only reduce cognitive

abilities, affect emotionality, and hinder the immune system, but it will also lead the person to make "bad" decisions, hence the importance of maintaining certain regularity and at least eight hours of sleep a day.

A behaviour to which some health professionals do not give due importance, considering that as long as they can stand they will attend to their position with the patients, which in some cases leads to extreme exhaustion, since the body has limited resources and has to recover both in terms of food and rest.

An aspect that should not be neglected, and shifts should be organized that allow health personnel to continue fulfilling their functions as effectively as possible after a good night's sleep, since failing to do so would be putting the worker himself at risk in addition to increasing the possibility of making mistakes in those tasks he performs (@ElLiberalDiario, 2020) (see Illustration 40).

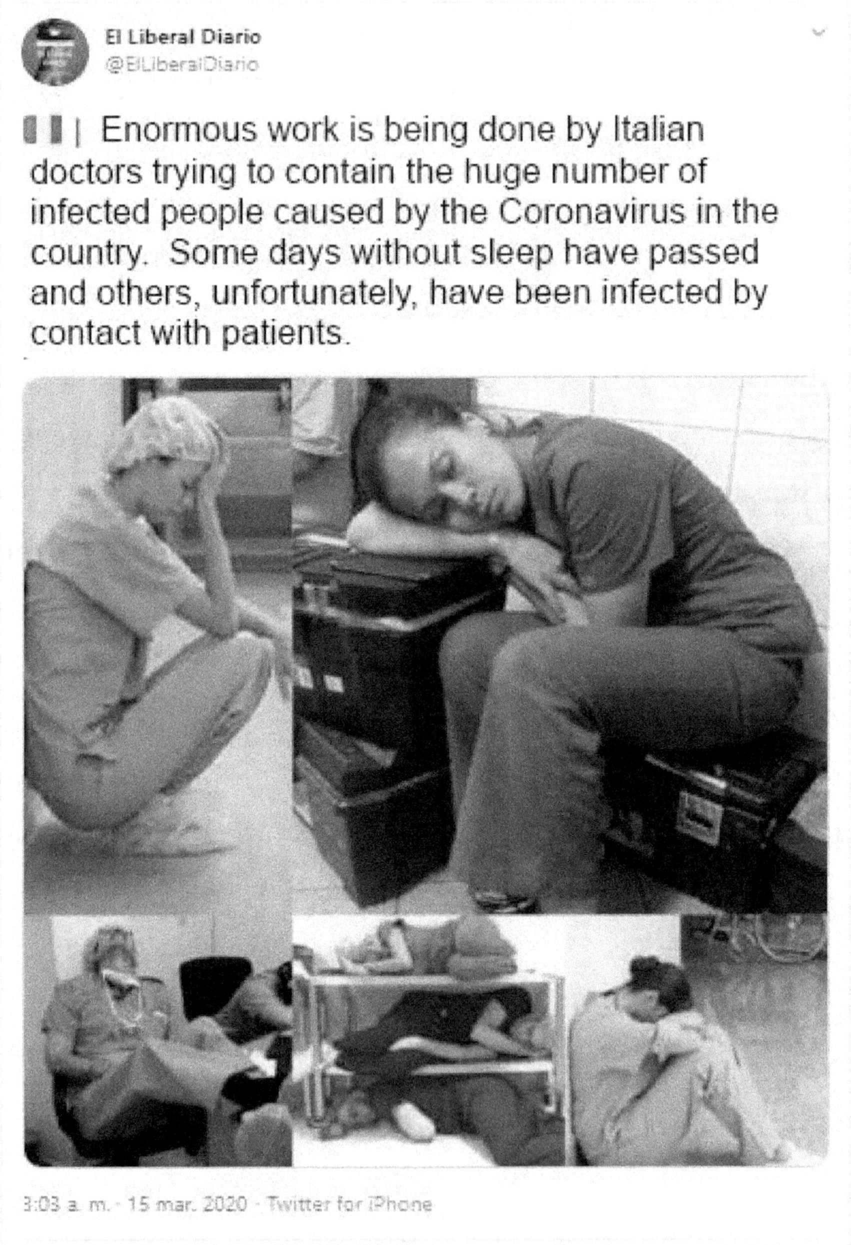

A Psychological Perspective of the Health Personnel in Times of Pandemic

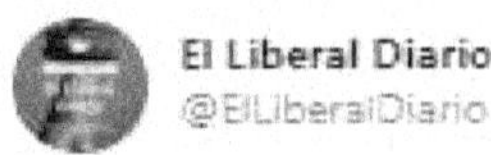

Illustration 40 Tweet Nurses Sleeping

Resilience in Healthcare Personnel

If we talk about the role of stress in the emotional sphere and its consequences on the body, we must refer to resilience, which has become a key concept in recent years in psychology as a way of handling with life.

Although the term resilience arose from the testimony of the survivors of the most extreme cases to which a person can be subjected, such as the survivors of the concentration camps in World War II, where it was analysed why some had survived and others had not, and among the survivors, why some managed to "rebuild their lives" and others were plunged into despair; when all had experienced the same horrors of war.

From this analysis and from testimonies such as that of Víctor Frankl, who developed logotherapy as a method of managing with these situations (Frankl, 2014) is where this kind of "formula" emerged to overcome any adversity, something that seems to be linked to the character of the person, but also with their way of thinking and seeing life.

Currently this concept is used in therapy, not only to care for people who have survived extreme situations, but to help them overcome the daily difficulties of life, aimed at reinforcing that resilience that everyone has inside.

Resilience is therefore a capacity that can be learned and developed, and that plays a fundamental role in protecting the person, since everyone is exposed to daily stress, but with an adequate development of resilience it is possible to learn to overcome difficulties that arise.

As indicated, healthcare personnel are exposed to high levels of stress, frustration and even suffer depressive symptoms, in addition to being exposed to burnout and aggressions by the patient and their family, for all the above it is necessary to understand the importance of resilience, which is presented as a protector against work stress, being defined as the ability of human beings to positively adapt to adverse situations, but what is the role of resilience in health personnel exposed to a pandemic?

This is what has been tried to find out by conducting research by Duke University School; together with Nanyang Technological University and the National Institute of Mental Health (Singapore) (Chang, Neo, & Fung, 2015).

To verify the role of resilience in the sphere of health in cases where they are subjected to higher levels of stress, the health personnel in charge of caring for the most contagious patients, and whose disease, due to its virulence, endangered, the life of anyone who is near without adequate protection, were selected; such is the case of nursing personnel who work in health care in the face of an epidemic like the one we are experiencing today.

Two investigations were carried out with these personnel and their families, in the first one involving 30 nurses aged between 30 to 56 years and an average of 10 years of service, who were given a semi-structured interview to verify their level of stress and their experience working with SARS (Severe Acute Respiratory Syndrome).

The responses were categorized according to most used terms by the nursing staff, which tried to define their way of thinking.

In the second study, 111 nurses and 78 of their relatives participated; to all of them were administered three tests, a scale of family resilience, one of personal resilience, and a third on their own perceived health status.

The results show in the first experiment, that these nurses were defined by a spirit of sacrifice towards their family, with a good capacity for emotional management, and strong religious convictions; factors all included in resilience.

Regarding the second study, the results obtained were analysed, with which it was possible to extract factors that were involved in resilience in the family environment, the value of solidarity in the family, the capacity for emotional regulation, the situation, and religious beliefs.

Comparing these results with the previous ones, it can be concluded that individual resilience can be predicted based on family resilience, that is, the person is capable of overcoming even the toughest difficulties, if they have been taught this in the family environment since they were little.

The contribution of the study is that it agrees that resilience is learned in the family environment; it is not that it prepares you for "the worst", but that in this area the necessary skills are developed to face the difficulties of daily life.

An education where Emotional Intelligence is developed, self-esteem is strengthened, and spiritual values are even cultivated, seem to be at the base of a future adult prepared to overcome even the most complicated difficulties that may arise in life.

But without going to extremes, these little ones, who grow up in a resilient family, will be better prepared to overcome the frustration of failure, seeing it as an opportunity to learn and grow, and thereby facilitating the path to success in what they proposed themselves to do.

Hence the importance that parents first, to learn

what resilience is and how it is cultivated, and then being able to express it and share it with their children in order to provide them with a better future.

References

@ 2010Asuka2010. (2020). Asuka on Twitter: 'Lidia nurse. We had to open ICUs on the run and without means. Paying with our health. Anxiety and fears. #BastaYa #NiHeroesNiMartires #MareaBlancaCoronavirus https://t.co/OWnhHKuphh '/ Twitter. Retrieved April 26 2020, from Twitter website: https://twitter.com/2010Asuka2010/status/1254506883475 542017

@Al_Jauregui_HVH. (2020). Albert Jauregui on Twitter: "Since I was a med student I have felt admiration for the #nursing collective. But in these days of crisis due to # COVID19 I have realized something else. Doctors cure patients, but #nursing are. Retrieved 20 April 2020, from Twitter website: https://twitter.com/Al_Jauregui_HVH/status/12508727983 49844484

@AUGC_Comunica. (2020). AUGC Guardia Civil on Twitter: "The Spanish Army sets up a field hospital in 48 hours with 5,500 beds at IFEMA." Retrieved 15 April 2020, from Twitter website: https://twitter.com/AUGC_Comunica/status/12420190388 19221505

@ Bastayamalaga2. (2020). Bastayamalaga on Twitter: 34 doctors have died in Spain from # Covid_19. We want to pay tribute to all of them. R.I.P. Retrieved 27 April 2020, from Twitter website:

https://twitter.com/Bastayamalaga2/status/125337839775
5060226

@CholutecaH. (2020). Choluteca Today on Twitter: "At least half the town could be infected by going to a funeral." Retrieved 19 April 2020, from Twitter website: https://twitter.com/CholutecaH/status/1251296885907881
984

@ColEnferMalaga. (2020). Col.EnfermeriaMalaga on Twitter: "@COPORIENTAL makes a free telephone number available to Andalusian health professionals for those who need psychological care. ☎ 851 00 520 # COEMálaga # nursesMálaga #COPAO https://t.co/mPJGuWz. Retrieved 26 April 2020, from Twitter website: https://twitter.com/ColEnferMalaga/status/124207246758
3250433

@CSIC. (2020). CSIC on Twitter: "The new #coronavirus is called SARS-CoV-2 and the disease it causes is COVID-19 (Coronavirus Disease 2019). The image, viruses of the Coronaviridae family, to which the new coronavirus belongs. (Photo taken by the virologist Luis En. Retrieved 4 April 2020, from https://twitter.com/CSIC/status/1236045267947970561

@ElLiberalDiario. (2020). El Liberal Diario on Twitter: Huge work is being done by Italian doctors trying to contain the huge number of infected people that caused the Coronavirus in the country. Days without sleep have passed some and others, unfortunately, have been inf. Retrieved 27 April 2020, from Twitter website: https://twitter.com/ElLiberalDiario/status/1239009235280

814080

@EPinternacional. (2020). International EP on Twitter: 'The plenary session of the European Parliament joins the applause for health workers against the #coronavirus https: //t.co/7WGSPF3aDR' / Twitter. Retrieved 21 April 2020, from Twitter website: https://twitter.com/EPinternacional/status/125086735524 6264320

@estrelladigital. (2020). Estrellaladigital.es on Twitter: "Madrid has begun the reincorporation of retired doctors under 70 years of age, the hiring of approved ones without a MIR, as well as students in the last year of Medicine and Nursing, among other measures https: // t . Retrieved 15 April 2020, from Twitter website: https://twitter.com/estrelladigital/status/12407562014466 12996

@ForcesOfOrder. (2020). Riot gear ?? on Twitter: 'Identified the man who painted" contagious rat "in a health care car ??? https://t.co/zz5TmtXq3W via @SquidAppES https://t.co/NR6toDdhwx '/ Twitter. Retrieved 18 April 2020, from Twitter website: https://twitter.com/FuerzasDelOrden/status/12512370477 52327171

@health. (2020). Sanidad on Twitter: 'Health system cancels congresses and meetings of health professionals due to the coronavirus @sanidadgob @salvadorilla #Coronavirus https: //t.co/57i6xfDxnV' / Twitter. Retrieved 15 April 2020, from Twitter website: https://twitter.com/isanidad/status/1235127894814396418

@JLo_RxM. (2020). Chogüe on Twitter: "Doctors and nurses have treated the infected with their usual hospital clothing. The situation and severity of this violently infectious or contagious virus forced them to be equipped with special clothing and esp. Retrieved 16 April 2020, from Twitter website: https://twitter.com/JLo_RxM/status/1249489139948326913

@Medicilio. (2020). Dr. Elena Casado Pineda on Twitter: "My name is Elena, I am an anaesthesiologist. There are more than 31,000 infected and more than 50 deaths. I am tired of working without resources and without respect. Of not seeing my family for fear of infecting them. I demand conditions. Retrieved 26 April 2020, from Twitter website: https://twitter.com/Medicilio/status/1254478344315441156

@moedetriana. (2020). Moe de Triana on Twitter: "The Netherlands wants to let its elderly die; France does not count deaths outside hospitals; Germany only numbers victims without previous pathologies ... because disgust does not understand borders either. Https: // t. co / V5N2H4. Retrieved 19 April 2020, from Twitter website: https://twitter.com/moedetriana/status/1243532765175349248

@Newtral. (2020). Newtral on Twitter: 'Masks, visors and even respirators. Thousands of people with 3D printers are trying to help healthcare workers by creating PPE material at home. https://t.co/lSVH3rjmMF https://t.co/peyLSQDWDP '/ Twitter. Retrieved 4 April 2020, from https://twitter.com/Newtral/status/1244782470580576257

@OMC_Espana. (2020a). College Medical Organization #NiUnDiaMas on Twitter: 'WE INSIST #NiUnDiaMas? 25.000 infected health workers 15,45% of the total ➡https: //t.co/bkxW3GgS0V # Covid19 #coronavirus #sanitarios #medical #medical #NiUnTestDeMenos https://t.co/zQI3VfhUML '. Retrieved 18 April 2020, from Twitter website: https://twitter.com/OMC_Espana/status/12490683402508 49280

@OMC_Espana. (2020b). Colegial Medical Organization #NiUnDiaMas on Twitter: 'The @Police supports threatened health workers and warns of possible criminal conduct https://t.co/oKVLnALNea #cuidaraquienesnoscuidan' / Twitter. Retrieved 18 April 2020, from Twitter website: https://twitter.com/OMC_Espana/status/12510562902243 73763

@psiquiatriacom. (2020). Psiquiatria.com on Twitter: 'I told him: "Everything will be fine, "and I failed him. I went down to the street to cry 'https: //t.co/sIlL0bh9YE https: //t.co/0CjArDWSqc' / Twitter. Retrieved 26 April 2020, from Twitter website: https://twitter.com/psiquiatriacom/status/1248177603313307649

@radio_angelica. (2020). Radio Angélica 99.7 on Twitter: "From the appearance of the first cases of coronavirus in December 2019, through the declaration of a pandemic by the WHO to widely exceed the barrier of one million infected, the new SARS-CoV-2 put the health system in check. . Retrieved 15 April 2020, from Twitter website: https://twitter.com/radio_angelica/status/12496747909836 55427

@radioyskl.   (2020). YSKL Radio on Twitter: "World Health Organization (WHO) Director Tedros Adhanom Ghebreyesus announced that the coronavirus has been renamed 'COVID-19'. An abbreviation of the disease that killed more than 1,000 people. La p. Retrieved 4 April 2020, from
https://twitter.com/radioyskl/status/12272967559869030 40

@Renzo_Utili.   (2020). Renzo on Twitter: '???   ITALY isolates 16 million people in rigid Quarantine, no one will be able to leave or enter only for very urgent reasons: map https://t.co/jOCVj3DtrS '/ Twitter. Retrieved 4 April 2020, from
https://twitter.com/Renzo_Utili/status/1236620725018116 101

@shildalys. (2020). ᏟhildalyᏟ on Twitter: "#coronoavirus
January 24, 2020: #China quarantines 8 more cities in Hubei province, trapping 35 million residents in their cities. Until now, 2019-nCoV has killed 26 patients, all in China. In. Retrieved 4 April 2020, from https://twitter.com/shildalys/status/1220867654560468998

@UNICEF_CLM.   (2020). UNICEF ComitéCLM on Twitter: 'Nurses, doctors, assistants, orderlies ... The longest applause in the world for all health workers THANK YOU!   https://t.co/oW4F45T1em '/ Twitter.

Retrieved 11 April 2020, from Twitter website:
https://twitter.com/UNICEF_CLM/status/1248309973148
467202

Abarca Cidon, J. (2020a). Good morning. We continue
with our chronicles of the war against the CV in HM
hospitals. LinkedIn. Retrieved 18 April 2020, from
LinkedIn website: https://www.linkedin.com/posts/juan-
abarca-cidon-b7b72122_buenos-dias-seguimos-con-
nuestras-cronicas-activity-6645896014756753409-HbNs/

Abarca Cidon, J. (2020b). Good morning, Sunday March
15 LinkedIn. Retrieved 18 April 2020, from LinkedIn
website: https://www.linkedin.com/posts/juan-abarca-
cidon-b7b72122_buenos-dias-del-domingo-15-de-marzo-
ayer-activity-6644846287227355136-1R6W/

Abarca Cidon, J. (2020c). Report of the war against the
coronavirus in HM in Madrid on March 11, 2020 LinkedIn.
Retrieved 18 April 2020, from LinkedIn website:
https://www.linkedin.com/posts/juan-abarca-cidon-
b7b72122_parte-de-guerra-contra-el-coronavirus-en-
activity-6643392899729891328-dITO/

It covers Cidon, J. (2020d). Report of the war against the
coronavirus in HM hospitals on March 12. LinkedIn.
Retrieved 18 April 2020, from LinkedIn website:
https://www.linkedin.com/posts/juan-abarca-cidon-
b7b72122_parte-de-guerra-contra-el-coronavirus-en-
activity-6643717774260609024-6Af1/

It covers Cidon, J. (2020e). Report of the war against the
CV of HM Hospitals from 1-04 LinkedIn. Retrieved 18

April 2020, from LinkedIn website: https://www.linkedin.com/posts/juan-abarca-cidon-b7b72122_parte-de-guerra-contra-el-cv-de-hm-hospitales-activity-6650969737582923776-5iT8 /

It covers Cidon, J. (2020f). Report of the war against the CV of 04/07 at HM Hospitals. LinkedIn. Retrieved 18 April 2020, from LinkedIn website: https://www.linkedin.com/posts/juan-abarca-cidon-b7b72122_parte-de-guerra-contra-el-cv-del-07-04-en-activity-6653145817328812032 -sX03 /

It includes Cidon, J. (2020g). Report of the war against the CV of March 25 in HM hospitals LinkedIn. Retrieved 18 April 2020, from LinkedIn website: https://www.linkedin.com/posts/juan-abarca-cidon-b7b72122_parte-de-guerra-contra-el-cv-del-25-de-marzo-activity-6648433954376433664 -uGz9 /

It covers Cidon, J. (2020h). Report of war against the CV of 27-03 LinkedIn. Retrieved 18 April 2020, from LinkedIn website: https://www.linkedin.com/posts/juan-abarca-cidon-b7b72122_parte-de-guerra-contra-el-cv-del-27-03-un-activity-6649167955412172800 -rwck /

It covers Cidon, J. (2020i). Report of the war against the CV of Monday 23-03 LinkedIn. Retrieved 18 April 2020, from LinkedIn website: https://www.linkedin.com/posts/juan-abarca-cidon-b7b72122_parte-de-guerra-contra-el-cv-del-lunes-23-activity-6647702326834540545-ZPcn /

Abarca Cidon, J. (2020j). Report of the war against the CV in HM hospitals from 12-04 LinkedIn. Retrieved 18 April

2020, from LinkedIn website:
https://www.linkedin.com/posts/juan-abarca-cidon-
b7b72122_parte-de-guerra-contra-el-cv-en-hm-hospitales-
activity-6654981161456140288-DOkf /

It covers Cidon, J. (2020k). Report of the war against the
CV at HM Hospitals on 04-16. Retrieved 18 April 2020,
from LinkedIn website:
https://www.linkedin.com/posts/juan-abarca-cidon-
b7b72122_parte-de-guerra-contra-el-cv-en-hm-hospitales-
activity-6656407723212701696-s0la /

It covers Cidon, J. (2020l). Report of the war of HM
Hospitals against the CV of 04-13 LinkedIn. Retrieved 18
April 2020, from LinkedIn website:
https://www.linkedin.com/posts/juan-abarca-cidon-
b7b72122_parte-de-guerra-de-hm-hospitales-contra-
activity-6655318834830024704-CLiL/

It covers Cidon, J. (2020m). One more day in the war
against the CV in HM. Possibly today 03-17 LinkedIn.
Retrieved 18 April 2020, from LinkedIn website:
https://www.linkedin.com/posts/juan-abarca-cidon-
b7b72122_un-dia-mas-en-la-guerra-contra-el-cv-en-hm-
activity -6645528471470776320-EDU0 /

Alexi, N. A., & Kathleen A. Moore. (2016). Seeking help
for mental illness: A qualitative study among Greek-
Australians and Anglo-Australians. Hellenic Journal of
Psychology, 13 (1), 1–12.
https://doi.org/10.13140/RG.2.2.16012.87687

Angelidis, A., Solis, E., Lautenbach, F., van der Does, W.,

& Putman, P. (2019). I'm going to fail! Acute cognitive performance anxiety increases threat-interference and impairs WM performance. PLoS ONE, 14 (2). https://doi.org/10.1371/journal.pone.0210824

Azeem, D. S. M. (2013). Conscientiousness, Neuroticism and Burnout among Healthcare Employees. International Journal of Academic Research in Business and Social Sciences, 3 (7). https://doi.org/10.6007/ijarbss/v3-i7/68

Baldonedo-Mosteiro, M., Almeida, M. C. dos S., Baptista, P. C. P., Sánchez-Zaballos, M., Rodriguez-Diaz, F. J., & Mosteiro-Diaz, M. P. (2019). Burnout syndrome in Brazilian and Spanish nursing workers. Latin American Journal of Nursing, 27. https://doi.org/10.1590/1518-8345.2818.3192

Barkham, M., Bewick, B., Mullin, T., Gilbody, S., Connell, J., Cahill, J., Evans, C. (2013). The CORE-10: A short measure of psychological distress for routine use in the psychological therapies. Counselling and Psychotherapy Research, 13 (1), 3–13. https://doi.org/10.1080/14733145.2012.729069

Buelow, M. T., & Suhr, J. A. (2009, March 5). Construct validity of the Iowa gambling task. Neuropsychology Review, Vol. 19, pp. 102-114. https://doi.org/10.1007/s11065-009-9083-4

Cassady, J. C., & Johnson, R. E. (2002). Cognitive test anxiety and academic performance. Contemporary Educational Psychology, 27 (2), 270–295.

Chang, W. C., Neo, A. H. C., & Fung, D. (2015). In Search

of Family Resilience. Psychology, 06 (13), 1594-1607. https://doi.org/10.4236/psych.2015.613157

Colten, H. R., & Altevogt, B. M. (2006). Sleep disorders and sleep deprivation: An unmet public health problem. In Sleep Disorders and Sleep Deprivation: An Unmet Public Health Problem. https://doi.org/10.17226/11617

General Council of Nursing. (2019). Aggression Statistics. Retrieved 19 April 2020, from Web of the General Council of Nursing website: https://www.consejogeneralenfermeria.org/observatorio-enfermero/agresiones/estadistica-de-agresiones

Cortini, M., Pivetti, M., & Cervai, S. (2016). Learning Climate and Job Performance among Health Workers. A Pilot Study. Frontiers in Psychology, 7 (OCT), 1644. https://doi.org/10.3389/fpsyg.2016.01644

Derryberry, D., & Reed, M. A. (2002). Anxiety-related Attentional biases and their regulation by Attentional control. Journal of Abnormal Psychology, 111 (2), 225–236. https://doi.org/10.1037/0021-843X.111.2.225

Egloff, B., Schwerdtfeger, A., & Schmukle, S. C. (2005). Temporal stability of the Implicit Association Test-Anxiety. Journal of Personality Assessment, 84 (1), 82–88. https://doi.org/10.1207/s15327752jpa8401_14

Eurostat. (2020). Healthcare resource statistics - beds - Statistics Explained. Retrieved 16 April 2020, from Web Eurostat website: https://ec.europa.eu/eurostat/statistics-explained/index.php/Healthcare_resource_statistics_-

_beds

Frankl, V. E. (2014). The will to meaning: Foundations and applications of logotherapy. Penguin.

Garrie, A. J., Goel, S., & Forsberg, M. M. (2016). Medical Students 'Perceptions of Dementia after Participation in Poetry Workshop with People with Dementia. International Journal of Alzheimer's disease, 2016. https://doi.org/10.1155/2016/2785105

Greenwald, A. G., McGhee, D. E., & Schwartz, J. L. K. (1998). Measuring individual differences in implicit cognition: The implicit association test. Journal of Personality and Social Psychology, 74 (6), 1464–1480. https://doi.org/10.1037/0022-3514.74.6.1464

Health Consumer Powerhouse Ltd. (2018). Euro Health Consumer Index 2018. Retrieved 16 April 2020, from Web Health Consumer Powerhouse Ltd website: https://healthpowerhouse.com/publications/#200118

Heath, P. J., Seidman, A. J., Vogel, D. L., Cornish, M. A., & Wade, N. G. (2017). Help-seeking stigma among men in the military: The interaction of restrictive emotionality and distress. Psychology of Men and Masculinity, 18 (3), 193–197. https://doi.org/10.1037/men0000111

Henry, J. D., & Crawford, J. R. (2005). The short-form version of the Depression anxiety stress scales (DASS-21): Construct validity and normative data in a large non-clinical sample. British Journal of Clinical Psychology, 44 (2), 227–239. https://doi.org/10.1348/014466505X29657

Horne, J. (2012, November 1). Working throughout the

night: Beyond 'sleepiness' - impairments to critical decision making. Neuroscience and Biobehavioral Reviews, Vol. 36, pp. 2226–2231. https://doi.org/10.1016/j.neubiorev.2012.08.005

Horowitz, M., Wilner, N., & Alvarez, W. (1979). Impact of Event Scale: A measure of subjective stress. Psychosomatic Medicine, 41 (3), 209–218.

Hübner, G., Mohs, A., & Petersen, L. E. (2014). The Role of Attitude Strength in Predicting Organ Donation Behaviour by Implicit and Explicit Attitude Measures. Open Journal of Medical Psychology, 03 (05), 355–363. https://doi.org/10.4236/ojmp.2014.35037

Carlos III Health Institute. (2020). Situation of COVID-19 or Coronavirus in Spain. Retrieved 15 April 2020, from Web Instituto de Salud Carlos III website: https://covid19.isciii.es/

Iwata, N., Mishima, N., Shimizu, T., Mizoue, T., Fukuhara, M., Hidano, T., & Spielberger, C. D. (1998). Positive and negative affect in the factor structure of the State-Trait Anxiety Inventory for Japanese workers. Psychological Reports, 82 (2), 651–656. https://doi.org/10.2466/pr0.1998.82.2.651

Jung, K., Shavitt, S., Viswanathan, M., & Hilbe, J. M. (2014). Female hurricanes are deadlier than male hurricanes. Proceedings of the National Academy of Sciences of the United States of America, 111 (24), 8782–8787. https://doi.org/10.1073/pnas.1402786111

Junta de Andalucía. (2019). Draft Law on the recognition of authority of teachers. Retrieved 18 April 2020, from Web of the Junta de Andalucía website: https://www.juntadeandalucia.es/servicios/normas-elaboracion/detalle/171905.html

Khaleghparast, S., Joolaee, S., Maleki, M., Peyrovi, H., Ghanbari, B., & Bahrani, N. (2016). Visiting hour's policies in intensive care units: Exploring participants' views. International Journal of Medical Research \ & Health Sciences, 5 (5), 322–328.

Krauth, C., Stahmeyer, J. T., Petersen, J. J., Freytag, A., Gerlach, F. M., & Gensichen, J. (2014). Resource Utilization and Costs of Depressive Patients in Germany: Results from the Primary Care Monitoring for Depressive Patients Trial. Depression Research and Treatment, 6, 730–891. https://doi.org/10.1155/2014/730891

Lana, A., Baizán, E. M., Faya-Ornia, G., & López, M. L. (2015). Emotional intelligence and health risk behaviours in nursing students. Journal of Nursing Education, 54 (8), 464–467.

Maslach, C, & Jackson, S. (1997). Inventario "Burnout" by Maslach. In TEA Ediciones (Ed.), MBI- Inventario "Burnout" by Maslach. Madrid.

Maslach, Christina, & Jackson, S. E. (1981). The measurement of experienced burnout. Journal of Organizational Behaviour, 2 (2), 99–113. https://doi.org/10.1002/job.4030020205

WHO. (2020a). Hospital beds per 100 000 - European

Health Information Gateway. Retrieved 15 April 2020, from Web O.M.S. website: https://gateway.euro.who.int/en/indicators/hfa_476-5050-hospital-beds-per-100-000/visualizations/#id=34379

WHO. (2020b). Questions and Answers on Coronavirus Disease (COVID-19). Retrieved 18 April 2020, from Web de la O.M.S. website: https://www.who.int/es/emergencies/diseases/novel-coronavirus-2019/advice-for-public/q-a-coronaviruses

U.N. (2014). WHO and UNICEF are the most respected agencies in the world. Retrieved 20 March 2020, from UN News website: https://news.un.org/es/story/2014/05/1301751

O'Connor, M. L., & McFadden, S. H. (2010). Development and Psychometric Validation of the Dementia Attitudes Scale. International Journal of Alzheimer's Disease, 2010. https://doi.org/10.4061/2010/454218

Odriozola-González, P., Planchuelo-Gómez, Á. Irurtia-Muñiz, M. J., & Luis-García, R. de. (2020). Psychological symptoms of the outbreak of the COVID-19 crisis and confinement in the population of Spain. Pre-Print. https://doi.org/10.31234/OSF.IO/MQ4FG

OECD / European Observatory on Health Systems and Policies. (2019). Spain: National Health Profile 2019, State of Health in the EU. Retrieved from http://www.oecd.org/health/Country-

Poon, S. T. F. (2016). Identifying and Comparing Mystery

and Honesty as Emotional Branding Values in Brand Personality Design. International Journal of Recent Scientific Research, 7 (3), 9241–9248.

Putman, P., Verkuil, B., Arias-Garcia, E., Pantazi, I., & Van Schie, C. (2014). EEG theta / beta ratio as a potential biomarker for Attentional control and resilience against deleterious effects of stress on attention. Cognitive, Affective and Behavioural Neuroscience, 14 (2), 782–791. https://doi.org/10.3758/s13415-013-0238-7

Ross, V., Sankaranarayanan, A., Lewin, T. J., & Hunter, M. (2016). Mental health workers 'views about their suicide prevention role. Psychology, Community & Health, 5 (1), 1–15. https://doi.org/10.5964/pch.v5i1.174

Salovey, P., & Mayer, J. D. (1990). Emotional Intelligence. Imagination, Cognition and Personality, 9 (3), 185–211. https://doi.org/10.2190/DUGG-P24E-52WK-6CDG

Selye, H. (1946). The General Adaptation Syndrome and the Diseases of Adaptation. The Journal of Clinical Endocrinology & Metabolism, 6 (2), 117–230. https://doi.org/10.1210/jcem-6-2-117

Smith, J. A., & Shinebourne, P. (2012). Interpretative phenomenological analysis. American Psychological Association.

Spielberger, C. D., Gorsuch, R. L., & Lushene, R. E. (1970). Manual for the State-Trait Anxiety Inventory.

Sriwijitalai, W., & Wiwanitkit, V. (2020). COVID-19 in forensic medicine unit personnel: Observation from Thailand. Journal of Forensic and Legal Medicine, 72,

101964. https://doi.org/10.1016/j.jflm.2020.101964

Thomson, W. (2014). The Head Stands Accused by the Heart! —Depression and Premature Death from Ischemic Heart Disease. Open Journal of Depression, 03 (02), 33–40. https://doi.org/10.4236/ojd.2014.32008

Van den Bos, R., Jolles, J. W., & Homberg, J. (2013, June 5). Social modulation of decision-making: A cross-species review. Frontiers in Human Neuroscience, Vol. 7, p. 301. https://doi.org/10.3389/fnhum.2013.00301

Vogel, D. L., Wade, N. G., & Haake, S. (2006). Measuring the self-stigma associated with seeking psychological help. Journal of Counselling Psychology, 53 (3), 325–337. https://doi.org/10.1037/0022-0167.53.3.325

Werneke, U., Goldberg, D. P., Yalcin, I., & Üstün, B. T. (2000). The stability of the factor structure of the general health questionnaire. Psychological Medicine, 30 (4), 823–829. https://doi.org/10.1017/S0033291799002287

Wester, S. R., Vogel, D. L., O'Neil, J. M., & Danforth, L. (2012). Development and evaluation of the Gender Role Conflict Scale Short Form (GRCS-SF). Psychology of Men and Masculinity, 13 (2), 199–210. https://doi.org/10.1037/a0025550

World Meteorological Organization. (2020). Tropical Cyclone Naming. Retrieved 7 March 2020, from https://public.wmo.int/en/About-us/FAQs/faqs-tropical-cyclones/tropical-cyclone-naming

Wynants, L., Van Calster, B., Bonten, M. M. J., Collins, G.

S., Debray, T. P. A., De Vos, M.,... van Smeden, M. (2020). Prediction models for diagnosis and prognosis of covid-19 infection: systematic review and critical appraisal. BMJ (Clinical Research Ed.), 369, m1328. https://doi.org/10.1136/bmj.m1328

Conclusions

With this work we have tried to present clearly and concisely the experience of health personnel when they have to face adversity, such as the current health crisis, with special emphasis on psychological aspects, since they will be subjected to high stress levels, an aspect that, together with personality factors, can facilitate the appearance of mental health problems.

Likewise, information is provided on the measures for the prevention of this type of problem, such as those adopted by the Official Associations of Psychologists, as well as the importance of resilience at this time.

Finally, take the opportunity to thank the work they do, essential and fundamental to be able to face and overcome a situation as serious as a pandemic, through a heartfelt tribute to the health personnel who have lost their lives while trying to save that of others (@ Bastayamalaga2, 2020) (see Illustration 41).

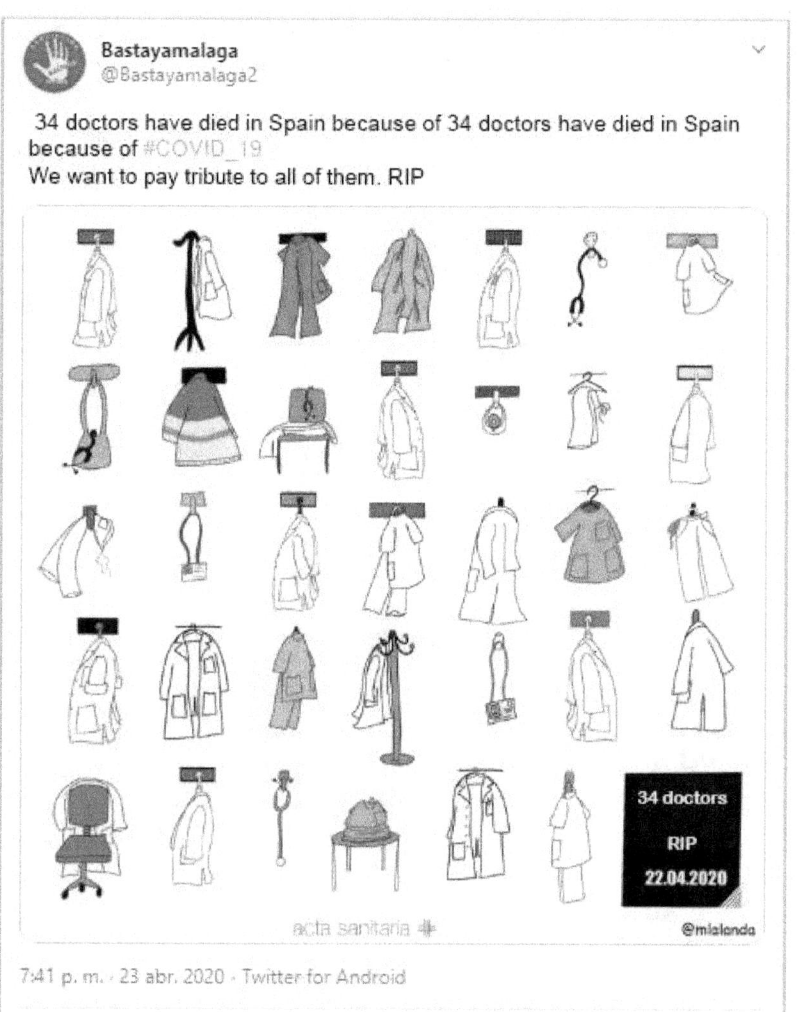

Illustration 41 Tweet Tribute to Doctors